# Medical
# Coding Workbook
## for Physician Practices and Facilities

## 2011-2012 Edition

*Cynthia Newby, CPC, CPC-P*

**Principal, Chestnut Hill Enterprises, Inc.**

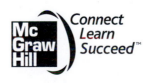

McGraw Hill

*Connect*
*Learn*
*Succeed*™

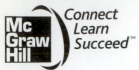

MEDICAL CODING WORKBOOK FOR PHYSICIAN PRACTICES AND FACILITIES
2011–2012 EDITION

Published by McGraw-Hill, a business unit of The McGraw-Hill Companies, Inc., 1221 Avenue of the
Americas, New York, NY, 10020. Copyright © 2012 by The McGraw-Hill Companies, Inc. All rights
reserved. Previous editions © 2002, 2005, 2006, 2008, and 2010. No part of this publication may be
reproduced or distributed in any form or by any means, or stored in a database or retrieval system,
without the prior written consent of The McGraw-Hill Companies, Inc., including, but not limited to,
in any network or other electronic storage or transmission, or broadcast for distance learning.

♲ Some ancillaries, including electronic and print components, may not be available to customers
outside the United States.

This book is printed on acid-free paper.

Printed in the United States of America.

4 5 6 7 8 9 0 QDB/QDB 1 0 9 8 7 6 5 4 3 2

ISBN      978-0-07-337488-8
MHID      0-07-337488-1

Vice president/Editor in chief: *Elizabeth Haefele*
Vice president/Director of marketing: *John E. Biernat*
Publisher: *Kenneth S. Kasee Jr.*
Senior sponsoring editor: *Natalie J. Ruffatto*
Director of development: *Sarah Wood*
Managing developmental editor: *Michelle L. Flomenhoft*
Developmental editor: *Raisa Priebe Kreek*
Executive marketing manager: *Roxan Kinsey*
Lead digital product manager: *Damian Moshak*
Director, Editing/Design/Production: *Jess Ann Kosic*
Project manager: *Marlena Pechan*
Buyer II: *Kara Kudronowicz*
Senior designer: *Srdjan Savanovic*
Media project manager: *Brent dela Cruz*
Media project manager: *Cathy L. Tepper*
Typeface: *11/13 Berkeley*
Compositor: *Aptara®, Inc.*
Printer: *Quad/Graphics*
Cover credit: © Devon Ford and Michael Glascott

The Internet addresses listed in the text were accurate at the time of publication. The inclusion of a
Web site does not indicate an endorsement by the authors or McGraw-Hill, and McGraw-Hill does not
guarantee the accuracy of the information presented at these sites. www.mhhe.com.

CPT five-digit codes, nomenclature, and other data are copyright © 2010, American Medical
Association. All rights reserved. No fee schedules, basic unit, relative values, or related listings are
included in CPT. The AMA assumes no liability for the data contained herein.

CPT codes are based on CPT 2011.

HCPCS codes are based on HCPCS 2011.

ICD-9-CM codes are based on ICD-9-CM 2011.

# Contents

TO THE STUDENT . . . . . . . . . . . . . . . . . . . . . . . . . . . . . . vii

TO THE INSTRUCTOR . . . . . . . . . . . . . . . . . . . . . . . . . . . vii

**PART 1**   **ICD-9-CM** . . . . . . . . . . . . . . . . . . . . . . . . . . . . . . 1

INTRODUCING ICD-10-CM . . . . . . . . . . . . . . . . . . . . . . . . . . . . . . . 2

LOCATING CORRECT CODES . . . . . . . . . . . . . . . . . . . . . . . . . . . . . . 2

APPLYING CODING GUIDELINES . . . . . . . . . . . . . . . . . . . . . . . . . . . . 3

V CODES (V01–V89)
Coding Tip: V Codes—Primary or Supplementary . . . . . . . . . . . . . . . . 5

E CODES (E000–E999)
Coding Tip: E Codes—A Supplementary Classification . . . . . . . . . . . 7

INFECTIOUS AND PARASITIC DISEASES (001–139)
Coding Tip: "Includes" Notes . . . . . . . . . . . . . . . . . . . . . 9

NEOPLASMS (140–239)
Coding Tip: The Neoplasm Table . . . . . . . . . . . . . . . . . . . . . . . 11

ENDOCRINE, NUTRITIONAL, AND METABOLIC DISEASES,
AND IMMUNITY DISORDERS (240–279)
Coding Tip: The Highest Level of Specificity—
Fourth and Fifth Digits . . . . . . . . . . . . . . . . . . . . . . . . . . . . . 13

DISEASES OF THE BLOOD AND BLOOD-FORMING ORGANS (280–289)
Coding Tip: The Colon and the Brace in the Tabular List . . . . . . . . . 15

MENTAL DISORDERS (290–319)
Coding Tip: The Abbreviations NEC and NOS . . . . . . . . . . . . . . . 17

DISEASES OF THE NERVOUS SYSTEM AND SENSE ORGANS (320–389)
Coding Tip: "Code First Underlying Disease" Instruction . . . . . . . . . 19

### DISEASES OF THE CIRCULATORY SYSTEM (390–459)
Coding Tip: "Excludes" Notes . . . . . . . . . . . . . . . . . . . . . . . . . . . . 21
Coding Tip: Hypertension . . . . . . . . . . . . . . . . . . . . . . . . . . . . . 23

### DISEASES OF THE RESPIRATORY SYSTEM (460–519)
Coding Tip: Chronic versus Acute Conditions . . . . . . . . . . . . . . 25

### DISEASES OF THE DIGESTIVE SYSTEM (520–579)
Coding Tip: Combination Codes . . . . . . . . . . . . . . . . . . . . . . . . . 27

### DISEASES OF THE GENITOURINARY SYSTEM (580–629)
Coding Tip: "Use Additional Code" Instruction . . . . . . . . . . . . . . 29

### COMPLICATIONS OF PREGNANCY, CHILDBIRTH, AND THE PUERPERIUM (630–679)
Coding Tip: Mothers' Conditions . . . . . . . . . . . . . . . . . . . . . . . . 31

### DISEASES OF THE SKIN AND SUBCUTANEOUS TISSUE (680–709)
Coding Tip: Notes at the Beginning of a Chapter . . . . . . . . . . . . . 33

### DISEASES OF THE MUSCULOSKELETAL SYSTEM AND CONNECTIVE TISSUE (710–739)
Coding Tip: Fifth-Digit Subclassifications by Site . . . . . . . . . . . . . 35

### CONGENITAL ANOMALIES (740–759)
Coding Tip: Congenital Anomalies and Patients' Ages . . . . . . . . . . 37

### CERTAIN CONDITIONS ORIGINATING IN THE PERINATAL PERIOD (760–779)
Coding Tip: Infants' Conditions . . . . . . . . . . . . . . . . . . . . . . . . . 39

### SYMPTOMS, SIGNS, AND ILL-DEFINED CONDITIONS (780–799)
Coding Tips: High Blood Pressure; HIV Codes . . . . . . . . . . . . . . . 41

### INJURY AND POISONING (800–999)
Coding Tips: Open versus Closed Fractures; Burns . . . . . . . . . . . . 43
Coding Tip: Poisoning versus Adverse Effects . . . . . . . . . . . . . . . 46
Coding Tip: Late Effects . . . . . . . . . . . . . . . . . . . . . . . . . . . . . . 47

### CODING QUIZ: ICD-9-CM . . . . . . . . . . . . . . . . . . . . . . . . . . . 49

## PART 2    CPT AND HCPCS . . . . . . . . . . . . . . . . . . . . . . . .55

### LOCATING CORRECT CODES . . . . . . . . . . . . . . . . . . . . . . . . . 56

### APPLYING CODING GUIDELINES . . . . . . . . . . . . . . . . . . . . . . 58

### MODIFIERS
Coding Tip: Bilateral and Unilateral Codes . . . . . . . . . . . . . . . . . 59

### EVALUATION AND MANAGEMENT (99201–99499) . . . . . . . . . . . 61
Coding Tips: Reimbursement for Consultations Depends on the Payer;
Problems Treated during Preventive Medicine Service . . . . . . . . . . 64

**ANESTHESIA SECTION (00100–01999)**
Coding Tip: Anesthesia Modifiers and Qualifying
Circumstances Codes . . . . . . . . . . . . . . . . . . . . . . . . . . . . . . . . . . . . 67

**SURGERY SECTION** . . . . . . . . . . . . . . . . . . . . . . . . . . . . . . . . . . . . . **69**

**INTEGUMENTARY SYSTEM (10040–19499)**
Coding Tip: Codes for Add-On Procedures . . . . . . . . . . . . . . . . . . . 71

**MUSCULOSKELETAL SYSTEM (20000–29999)**
Coding Tip: Package Codes and Global Periods . . . . . . . . . . . . . . . 73

**RESPIRATORY SYSTEM (30000–32999)**
Coding Tip: Codes That Include Conscious Sedation . . . . . . . . . . . 77

**CARDIOVASCULAR SYSTEM (33010–37799)**
Coding Tip: Radiological Supervision and Interpretation . . . . . . . . . 79

**HEMIC AND LYMPHATIC SYSTEMS; MEDIASTINUM AND DIAPHRAGM (38100–39599)**
Coding Tip: Surgical Procedures Include Diagnostic Procedures . . . . 83

**DIGESTIVE SYSTEM (40490–49999)**
Coding Tip: Separate Procedures . . . . . . . . . . . . . . . . . . . . . . . . . . 85

**URINARY SYSTEM (50010–53899)**
Coding Tip: Procedures Performed
Using Various Techniques or Approaches . . . . . . . . . . . . . . . . . . . . . 87

**MALE GENITAL SYSTEM; INTERSEX SURGERY (54000–55980)**
Coding Tip: Biopsies . . . . . . . . . . . . . . . . . . . . . . . . . . . . . . . . . . . . 89

**FEMALE GENITAL SYSTEM; MATERNITY CARE AND DELIVERY (56405–59899)**
Coding Tip: The Obstetric Package . . . . . . . . . . . . . . . . . . . . . . . . . 91

**ENDOCRINE SYSTEM; NERVOUS SYSTEM (60000–64999)**
Coding Tip: Procedures Exempt from the -51 Modifier . . . . . . . . . . . 93

**EYE AND OCULAR ADNEXA; AUDITORY SYSTEM; OPERATING MICROSCOPE (65091–69990)**
Coding Tip: Operating Microscope . . . . . . . . . . . . . . . . . . . . . . . . . 95

**RADIOLOGY SECTION (70010–79999)**
Coding Tip: Unlisted Procedures and Special Reports . . . . . . . . . . . 97

**PATHOLOGY AND LABORATORY SECTION (80047–89398)**
Coding Tip: Panels . . . . . . . . . . . . . . . . . . . . . . . . . . . . . . . . . . . . . . 99

**MEDICINE SECTION (90281–99607)**
Coding Tip: Injections . . . . . . . . . . . . . . . . . . . . . . . . . . . . . . . . . . 101
Coding Tip: Cardiac Catheterization . . . . . . . . . . . . . . . . . . . . . . . 103

**CATEGORY II CODES (0001F–7025F)**
Coding Tip: Category II Code Updates . . . . . . . . . . . . . . . . . . . . . . 105

**CATEGORY III CODES (0019T-0259T)** . . . . . . . . . . . . . . . . . . . . . . . **107**
Coding Tip: Category III Code Updates . . . . . . . . . . . . . . . . . . . . . 107

**HEALTH CARE COMMON PROCEDURE CODING SYSTEM (HCPCS)** . . . . . . . . . 109

Coding Tip: Locating Correct HCPCS Codes . . . . . . . . . . . . . . . 110

Coding Tip: ABN Modifiers . . . . . . . . . . . . . . . . . . . . . 110

**HCPCS LEVEL II NATIONAL CODES AND MODIFIERS** . . . . . . . . . . . . . . . . 111

**CODING QUIZ: CPT AND HCPCS** . . . . . . . . . . . . . . . . . . . . . . . 113

**PART 3**   **PHYSICIAN AND FACILITY CODING LINKAGE AND COMPLIANCE** . . . . . . . . . . . . . 121

**CODE LINKAGE** . . . . . . . . . . . . . . . . . . . . . . . . . . . 123

**COMMON CODING ERRORS** . . . . . . . . . . . . . . . . . . . . . . 123

**CODING COMPLIANCE** . . . . . . . . . . . . . . . . . . . . . . . . 124

**SECTION 1**

Coding Tip: Verifying Linkage . . . . . . . . . . . . . . . . . . . 125

**SECTION 2**

Coding Tip: Selecting the Primary Diagnosis . . . . . . . . . . . . 127

**SECTION 3**

Coding Tip: Reporting Chronic or Undiagnosed Conditions . . . . . . 129

**SECTION 4**

Coding Tip: Using V and E Codes for a Clear Picture
of an Encounter . . . . . . . . . . . . . . . . . . . . . . . . . . 131

**SECTION 5**

Coding Tip: Avoiding Unspecified Diagnostic Codes . . . . . . . . . 133

**SECTION 6**

Coding Tip: Reporting Surgical Diagnoses and Complications . . . . . 135

**SECTION 7**

Coding Tips: Reporting Bundled (Global) Procedures and Laboratory
Panels; Using Correct Code Sets . . . . . . . . . . . . . . . . . . 137

**SECTION 8**

Coding Tips: ICD-9-CM Official Guidelines for Coding and Reporting;
ICD-9-CM Volume 3 . . . . . . . . . . . . . . . . . . . . . . . . . 139

**CODING QUIZ: COMPLIANCE** . . . . . . . . . . . . . . . . . . . . . 149

**APPENDIX A**   **ICD-9-CM OFFICIAL GUIDELINES FOR CODING AND REPORTING OUTPATIENT SERVICES** . . . . . . . . . . . . 153

**APPENDIX B**   **CPT MODIFIERS** . . . . . . . . . . . . . . . . . . . 155

BLANK ANSWER SHEETS FOR QUIZZES . . . . . . . . . . . . . . . 157–159

# To the Student

Expertise in working with the HIPAA-mandated code sets found in ICD-9-CM and CPT/HCPCS is the baseline for correct coding. The diagnosis and procedure codes that physician practices and hospitals report to payers must be properly assigned based on current classifications. Equally important is knowing how to assign and report codes in compliance with government and other regulations such as HIPAA. To avoid potential billing fraud, the diagnoses on each medical insurance claim must support the medical necessity of the procedures. In addition to this code linkage, the reported services and procedures must be correctly documented in the patient medical record.

With many thousands of diagnosis and procedure codes to select from, however, developing coding expertise cannot be based on memorization or on trial and error! Rather, coders must understand the structure and conventions used in ICD-9-CM and CPT/HCPCS, and know the guidelines for applying the codes. Coders also need to know the principles that underlie rules and regulations for compliant claims.

*Medical Coding Workbook for Physician Practices and Facilities* builds coding expertise by providing extensive practice in code selection. It is designed to be used in conjunction with ICD-9-CM, Volumes 1 and 2, and with CPT/HCPCS. ICD-9-CM Volume 3 is needed for Section 8 of Part 3. A medical dictionary and other medical references will also be helpful as you work through the coding exercises.

The workbook has three sections: Part 1, ICD-9-CM; Part 2, CPT and HCPCS; and Part 3, Physician and Facility Coding Linkage and Compliance. The exercises in the parts follow the structure of the coding references. Each set of exercises also presents Coding Tips to extend your knowledge of coding principles.

Because of the importance of correct coding, many medical coders seek certification as professional coders from organizations such as the American Academy of Professional Coders and the American Health Information Management Association. Certification examinations are taken after the coder has had both coding education and work experience. The Coding Quizzes in *Medical Coding Workbook for Physician Practices and Facilities* introduce you to the format of these exams and are useful in helping you build coding skill.

# To the Instructor

*Medical Coding Workbook for Physician Practices and Facilities* is designed for use by students who have a basic understanding of medical coding from introductory instruction. For example, the McGraw-Hill text *Medical Insurance* is designed for medical insurance courses and devotes three chapters to physician practice coding. In the text, students learn the structure and conventions of ICD-9-CM and CPT/HCPCS and the correct process for selecting codes, as well as types of coding errors to be avoided.

# New for the 2011–2012 Edition

Key content changes include:

- Free 14-day access for CodeitRightOnline™.
- All codes and conventions updated for the 2011 code sets: ICD-9-CM, CPT, HCPCS.

Explanations and/or exercises added for new topics:

- BMI ranges in adults
- Text messaging accident, swine flu
- CPT new structure that features resequencing of codes
- New organization of CPT Evaluation and Management section codes
- CMS nonpayment of CPT E/M consultation codes
- New guideline for reporting overlapping pathology/laboratory panels
- Reference to the AMA CPT vaccine product code updates website
- New ABN modifiers
- Updated Official Guidelines for Coding and Reporting Outpatient Services
- Brief introduction to ICD-10-CM and note on ICD-10-PCS

Answers to the exercises in this workbook are available for instructors using *Medical Coding Workbook for Physician Practices and Facilities* at the book's Online Learning Center, www.mhhe.com/codingwkbk6e. It is also posted to the Online Learning Center for Valerius, *Medical Insurance* at www.mhhe.com/valerius5e. Your McGraw-Hill sales representative can provide you with access.

The technical reviewers acknowledged on page xi offered invaluable assistance in reviewing the exercises, answers, and coding tips for accuracy. The reviewers and I hope that we have been correct in our work. Any errors, however, are the author's responsibility. You are encouraged to report these to the publisher, so that corrections can be made.

# CodeitRightOnline™: Your Online Coding Tool

So that your students can gain experience with the use of an online coding tool, they will have access for a 14-day period to CodeitRightOnline, produced by Contexo Media, a division of Access Intelligence.

# Features

These are the general features that are offered with a subscription:

- **CodeitRightOnline Search**—The ability to find a CPT, HCPCS Level II, and ICD-9-CM code either using the Index or Tabular search sections, by code terminology, description, keyword, or code number to locate the correct code. Plus, the Single Search Feature allows you to locate all codes related to a particular term.
- **Fully customizable**—Provides note capability, LCD customization, personalized searches and fee schedules, and specialty-specific code sets.
- **Print Custom Coding Books**—Subscribers can create and print their own specialty-specific CPT, HCPCS, ICD-9-CM, and RVU books.

- **Coding Crosswalks**—Essential coding links from CPT codes to ICD-9-CM to HCPCS Level II codes and to Anesthesia codes.
- **Articles**—We have compiled articles from CMS, OIG, carriers, intermediaries, payers, and other government websites along with newsletter articles from AMA, AHA, Decision Health, Coding Institute, and others.
- **Plus**—LCD/NCD codes for a local state carrier, Medicare's payment policy indicators, and, of course, CPT®, HCPCS Level II, and ICD-9-CM codes with full descriptions and our Plain English Definitions.
- **ICD-10-CM/PCS Code Sets**—Helps you prepare for 2013 mandatory implementation with ICD-10-CM/PCS full code sets and descriptions.
- **NCCI Edits Validator™**—Validates codes to help you remain in compliance with the correct coding guidelines established by the Centers for Medicare & Medicaid Services (CMS).
- **Automatic Updates**—Ensures that CodeitRightOnline contains the most up-to-date, real-time information.
- **Build-A-Code™**—Allows students to build codes from the ground up, helping them understand how ICD-10 codes are constructed.
- **Click-A-Dex™**—Helps index searches for easy future reference.
- **Comprehensive Medicare Resource**—Contains local coverage determination (LCD) and national coverage determination (NCD) information, contact information for comprehensive list of Medicare providers, and information on how to bill for procedures allowed by Medicare's Physician Quality Reporting Initiative (PQRI) program.
- **ABC Codes and Descriptions**—Provide access to the alternative medicine codes you need to describe services, remedies, and/or supplies required during patient visits.

## Using the Online Coding Tool

Go to CodeitRightOnline to complete the steps needed to begin. The following screen will appear:

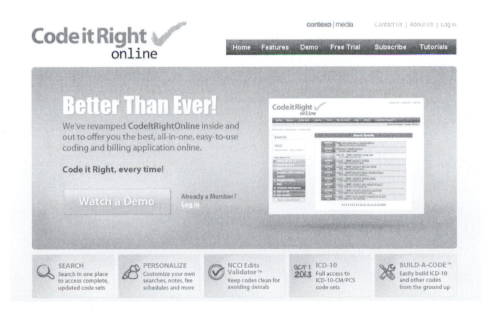

Click on the Free Trial tab at the top right-hand corner of the screen. On the page that appears, enter your name, e-mail address, school, phone, and address. Next, click on "Use account contact information" for your account administrator information, a one-time process that optimizes CodeitRightOnline for your particular location. Choose a username and password you will remember. Next, read the Terms and Conditions, including the AMA Agreement. After accepting these Terms and Conditions, click Continue. You will then receive an e-mail containing an activation link. Clicking on the link will activate your account. From that page, follow the "Click here" link to sign in with the account information you selected. This will take you to the Code-itRightOnline home page—you're in!

These actions set up your trial subscription. Now, to use the online coding tool to locate codes, click Search and select the appropriate code set. Next, choose the start point for your code search. For example, select ICD-9-CM Vol 1,2 and Vol 3 in the Show Results For box, enter the term *fracture,* and click Search. CodeitRightOnline will return a list of the various fracture entries for your selection. To see how it works, choose Fracture of Ribs, Closed and click the code number to review the Tabular List entry.

# Blackboard

McGraw-Hill Higher Education and Blackboard have teamed up. What does this mean for you?

1. **Your life, simplified.** Now you and your students can access McGraw-Hill's Connect™ and Create™ right from within your Blackboard course—all with one single sign-on. Say goodbye to the days of logging in to multiple applications.

2. **Deep integration of content and tools.** Not only do you get single sign-on with Connect™ and Create™, you also get deep integration of McGraw-Hill content and content engines right in Blackboard. Whether you're choosing a book for your course or building Connect™ assignments, all the tools you need are right where you want them—inside of Blackboard.

3. **Seamless Gradebooks.** Are you tired of keeping multiple gradebooks and manually synchronizing grades into Blackboard? We thought so. When a student completes an integrated Connect™ assignment, the grade for that assignment automatically (and instantly) feeds your Blackboard grade center.

4. **A solution for everyone.** Whether your institution is already using Blackboard or you just want to try Blackboard on your own, we have a solution for you. McGraw-Hill and Blackboard can now offer you easy access to industry leading technology and content, whether your campus hosts it, or we do. Be sure to ask your local McGraw-Hill representative for details.

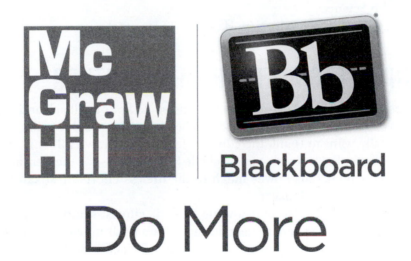

Do More

# Acknowledgments

Suggestions have been received from faculty and students throughout the country. This is vital feedback that is relied upon with each edition. Each of those who have offered comments and suggestions has our thanks.

The efforts of many people are needed to develop and improve a product. Among these people are the reviewers and consultants who point out areas of concern, cite areas of strength, and make recommendations for change. In this regard, the following people provided feedback that was enormously helpful in preparing the new edition.

- Toni L. Clough, Health Claim Adjuster, Umpqua Community College
- Carol T. Courtney, MS, CPC, OCS, Clark Community College
- Barbara L. Donnally, CPC, University of Rio Grande
- Amy Ensign, CMA (AAMA), RMA (AMT), Baker College of Clinton Township
- Amy E. Higgins, CPC, BA, Career College of Northern Nevada
- Traci Hotard, RHIA, SCL Technical College
- Fannie Sue Martin, CPC, YTI Career Institute
- Zetta McClain, NCICS, RMA, MBA, NCPT, Baker College of Auburn Hills
- Kimberly Rash, Associates, Applied Science, Gateway Community and Technical College
- Elaine M. Tuholski, CPC
- Stacey F. Wilson, CMA (AAMA), MT/PBT (ASCP), MHA, Cabarrus College of Health Sciences
- Amy L. Wood, CPC, Yale–New Haven (CT) Hospital

## ACKNOWLEDGMENTS FROM THE AUTHOR

To the students and instructors who use this book, your feedback and suggestions have made the Coding Workbook a better learning tool for all.

I especially want to thank the editorial team at McGraw-Hill—Liz Haefele, Natalie Ruffatto, Raisa Kreek, and Michelle Flomenhoft—for their enthusiastic support. This book's also owes much to the tireless efforts of Roxan Kinsey, Executive Marketing Manager.

The EDP staff was also outstanding in their efforts; senior designer Srdj Savanovic, Marlena Pechan, project manager, Kara Kudronowicz, buyer, Carrie Burger, photo research coordinator, and Brent Delacruz and Cathy Tepper, media project managers.

Thanks to this enthusiastic and dedicated team for making the revision process a seamless one!

*Cynthia Newby, CPC, CPC-P*

# Part 1 ICD-9-CM

The diagnostic codes used in the United States are based on the *International Classification of Diseases* (ICD). The ICD is a publication listing diseases and injuries with their three-digit codes according to a system maintained by the World Health Organization of the United Nations.

A United States version of the ninth edition of the ICD (ICD-9) was published in 1979. A committee of physicians from various organizations and specialties prepared this version, which is called the ICD-9's clinical modification and abbreviated as ICD-9-CM. It is used to code and classify morbidity data from patient medical records, physician practices, and surveys conducted by the National Center for Health Statistics (NCHS). The ICD is the classification used by the federal government to categorize mortality data from death certificates. Codes in the ICD-9-CM describe conditions and illnesses more precisely than do the World Health Organization's ICD-9 codes because they are intended to provide a more complete picture of patients' conditions.

ICD-9-CM is the HIPAA-mandated diagnosis code set. Updates, called the addenda, for the ICD-9-CM are released twice a year (October 1 and April 1) by NCHS and the Centers for Medicare and Medicaid Services (CMS). New codes are added and others are revised or deleted.

Under HIPAA, there is no grace period for implementing code changes. The new, correct codes must be used for all services performed on or after their effective date. Medical coders need to keep up with these changes and ensure that the codes in effect on the date of service are used.

Diagnostic coding in physician practices is based on Volumes 1 and 2 of the ICD-9-CM. The choice of the right code follows specific guidelines developed by a group made up of CMS advisors and participants from the American Hospital Association, the American Health Information Management Association, and NCHS. The guidelines cover what is to be coded and in what order the codes should be reported. These Official Guidelines for Coding and Reporting of patient services are reprinted in Appendix A on pages 153–154.

# Introducing ICD-10-CM

The tenth edition of the ICD was published by the World Health Organization in 1990. HHS, under a HIPAA Final Rule on January 16, 2009, mandated the adoption of this new diagnosis code set, called ICD-10-CM, as of October 1, 2013. This new code set, already used in many other countries, has been developed in order to provide many improvements to ICD-9-CM.

ICD-10-CM provides many more categories for disease and other health-related conditions and much greater flexibility for adding new codes in the future. It is a larger code set, having about 141,000 codes versus ICD-9-CM's approximately 13,000. It also offers a higher level of specificity and additional character and extensions for expanded detail. There are also many more codes that combine etiology and manifestations, poisoning and external cause, or diagnosis and symptoms. Medical coders who are knowledgeable users of ICD-9-CM will quickly learn to work efficiently with the new code set in 2013.

# Locating Correct Codes

Medical coders follow a series of steps to choose correct ICD-9-CM codes.

## Step 1.
### Analyze the Reason for the Encounter

The primary diagnosis—the main reason for the patient's encounter—is documented in the patient's medical record. It is the diagnosis, condition, problem, or other reason that the documentation shows is chiefly responsible for the services that are provided. This primary diagnosis provides the main term to be coded first. If other conditions or problems are pertinent or treated, they are also coded.

## Step 2.
### Locate the Term in the Alphabetic Index

The Alphabetic Index is then used to find the medical term that describes the patient's primary diagnosis. Each main term in the index is printed in boldface type and is followed by its code number. Below the main term, any subterms and their codes appear. Subterms may show the etiology of the disease—its cause or origin—or describe a particular type of disease or body site. Any supplementary terms are shown in parentheses after the main term. Supplementary terms are not essential to the selection of the correct code. They are included to help point to the correct term, but they do not have to appear in the physician's statement of the diagnosis. A "see" cross-reference after a main term means that another category must be used. "See also category" indicates that the additional listed categories should be reviewed. Notes beneath entries provide more information on selecting the correct code.

Many terms appear more than once in the Alphabetic Index. Often, the term in common use is listed, as well as the accepted medical terminology. Many eponyms—conditions (or procedures) named for persons or places—

appear. An eponym is usually listed both under that name and under the main term for the disease or syndrome.

Follow these guidelines to pick the correct main term:

- Use any supplementary terms in the diagnostic statement to help locate the main term.
- Read and follow any notes below the main term.
- Review the subterms to find the most specific match to the diagnosis.
- Read and follow any cross-references.
- Make note of a two-code (etiology and manifestation) indication and identify both codes that are required.

## Step 3.
## Verify the Code in the Tabular List

The medical coder next verifies the code for the medical term in the Tabular List of the ICD-9-CM. Diseases and injuries in the Tabular List are organized into chapters according to etiology or body system. Chapters are divided into sections that group related code categories. Within each section, there are three levels of codes:

1. A category is a three-digit code that covers a single disease or related condition.
2. A subcategory is a four-digit subdivision of a category. It provides a further breakdown of the disease to show its etiology, site, or manifestation.
3. A subclassification is a five-digit subdivision of a subcategory. Supplementary codes and appendixes cover other special situations.

Never code from only the Alphabetic Index. This practice causes coding errors. Always use the subclassification level—five digits—if available.

# Applying Coding Guidelines

The *Medical Coding Workbook for Physician Practices and Facilities* is designed to build your skill in applying ICD-9-CM coding guidelines. Each chapter of exercises begins with a *Coding Tip* that explains important diagnostic coding rules, processes, or information. Some of these tips apply just to the particular ICD-9-CM chapter in which you are studying them, and others apply globally when coding diseases and injuries. After completion of all the exercises in this part, you will know how to apply guidelines concerning

- V codes—primary or supplementary
- E codes—a supplementary classification
- "Includes" notes
- The neoplasm table
- The highest level of specificity—fourth and fifth digits
- The colon and the brace in the tabular list
- The abbreviations NEC and NOS
- "Code first underlying disease" instruction
- "Excludes" notes

- The hypertension table
- Combination codes
- "Use additional code" instruction
- Mothers' conditions
- Notes at the beginning of a chapter
- Fifth-digit subclassifications by site
- Congenital anomalies and patients' ages
- Infants' conditions
- High blood pressure
- HIV codes
- Open versus closed fractures
- Burns
- Poisoning versus adverse effects
- Late effects

# V Codes—Supplementary Classification of Factors Influencing Health Status and Contact with Health Services

## Codes V01–V89

V codes identify encounters for reasons other than illness or injury. V codes are used for four main types of encounters: (1) healthy patients who receive services other than treatments, such as annual checkups, immunizations, and normal childbirth; (2) patients with known conditions for which they are receiving chemotherapy, radiation therapy, and rehabilitation aftercare; (3) patients with a problem that is not currently affecting their health status but that should be noted, such as a family history of a disease; and (4) patients being evaluated before an operation.

---

### CODING TIP

#### V Codes—Primary or Supplementary

V codes are used as the primary code—that is, listed first—when healthy patients receive services, patients receive treatment for a current or resolving condition, and patients are evaluated preoperatively. Some V codes, however, are never primary. Rather, these codes are always supplementary—they are additional codes that are listed after a primary code for the encounter. A problem influencing a patient's health status that is not currently an illness or injury—such as a family history of a chronic disease—is an example of a supplementary V code. In this case, the patient's reason for the encounter is listed first, followed by a V code for the influencing factor.

---

### Provide the V code.

1. routine medical examination _____

2. exposure to tuberculosis _____

3. glaucoma screening _____

4. supervision of high-risk first pregnancy in a 15-year-old female _____

5. measles vaccination _____

6. admission for prophylactic removal of ovary _____

7. BMI of 46.9 in an adult patient _____

8. heart transplant (status post) _____

9. diaphragm fitting _____

10. contact with *E. coli* _____

## Provide the V code, and indicate whether it is a primary or a supplemental code.

11. preoperative cardiovascular examination _____

12. encounter for hospice care _____

13. health examination of preschool children _____

14. counseling for marital problems _____

15. supervision of normal first pregnancy _____

16. patient's parents are both deaf _____

17. history of allergy to dust _____

18. patient suspected of carrying hepatitis C _____

19. infection with penicillin-resistant microorganism _____

20. encounter for suture removal _____

## Select the V code for the following case studies.

21. A 55-year-old patient is new to the internist seeing him today for his annual physical. During the discussion regarding the patient's medical history, he mentions that his father and grandfather had polycystic kidney disease, and he has some concerns regarding his potential for developing the same problem. In addition to the diagnosis code for the annual physical, what other diagnosis code would be needed? _____

22. A 35-year-old pregnant patient has asked her obstetrician to perform an amniocentesis. She has no specific anomalies or genetic predispositions, but is concerned for the well-being of her baby. No specific condition was found during the amniocentesis. What diagnosis code is used for the amniocentesis? _____

23. After a serious accident 2 months ago, a patient's left eye was removed. The patient now returns for fitting of the artificial eye that will replace the eye that was removed. _____

24. After testing of his patient's sister, the nephrologist determines that the sister is an appropriate candidate to donate a kidney for her brother's kidney transplant. Today, she is admitted to hospital as a kidney donor. What diagnosis code is used for her hospital admission? _____

25. The patient has been seen by her gynecologist for close to 20 years, for her 3 pregnancies and a one-time abnormal pap smear. Today she is being seen for her annual routine pelvic exam. Which V code is appropriate?

_____

# E Codes—Supplementary Classification of External Causes of Injury and Poisoning

## Codes E000–E999

E (for external) codes classify injuries resulting from environmental events such as falls, fires, transportation accidents, accidental poisoning by a drug or other substances, and adverse effects, a patient's harmful reaction to the correct dosage of a drug (categories E930 to E949). The Table of Drugs and Chemicals that appears after the Alphabetic Index lists these agents alphabetically, and columns 2 through 6 contain the E codes for the situation: accidental, therapeutic, suicide attempt, assault, or undetermined use of the drug or chemical. The Alphabetic Index to External Causes of Injury and Poisoning that follows the Table of Drugs and Chemicals lists main terms for external causes—the accident, circumstance, event, or agent (drug or chemical) that caused the injury.

---

### CODING TIP

#### E Codes—A Supplementary Classification

External causes are not the primary diagnoses of patients' conditions, so E codes are never used alone. Instead, E codes always supplement a code that identifies the injury or condition itself. The primary diagnosis code is listed first, followed by the additional E code.

---

### Identify the E codes for the following substances in the Table of Drugs and Chemicals.

1. accidental poisoning by barbiturates _____

2. accidental poisoning by malathion _____

3. injury from ingesting oestriol _____

4. suicide attempt with aspirin _____

5. adverse effect from diphtheria vaccine _____

### Provide the E codes for the following descriptions.

6. accidental drowning after fall from water skis _____

7. fall from a window _____

8. sunstroke _____

9. bee sting _____

10. injury to driver in motor vehicle collision with a stalled car _____

11. exposure to radiation _____

12. burn caused by flames of gas grill in kitchen _____

13. railway passenger injured while boarding the train _____

14. adverse reaction to antiparkinsonism drug _____

15. accident due to text messaging while driving _____

## Provide both the primary code for the patient's diagnosis and the supplemental E code in the correct order.

16. allergic reaction to synthetic penicillin *Hint:* First code the allergic reaction and then code the adverse reaction to the therapeutic use. _____

17. fractured thumb on right hand resulting from a fall from a ladder _____

18. dermatitis due to an adverse reaction to antihistamine _____

19. patient tackled and knocked down during football game, suffers concussion with loss of consciousness for 20 minutes _____

20. coma caused by overdose of tranquilizers in suicide attempt _____

## Select the E code for the following case studies.

21. A patient was brought to the emergency department by ambulance after suffering a fractured left arm and left leg, with multiple soft tissue injuries. It was determined that the patient was the pilot of an airplane that had crashed during a forced landing._____

22. A patient was found unconscious at home, holding a bottle of glue, and a note was found indicating attempted suicide. _____

23. An elderly patient who recently had new dentures put in was talking excitedly on the phone while eating her lunch. The food became lodged in her esophagus, causing suffocation. _____

24. A patient who had recently moved to a new city was seen by her new internist for the first time due to an ongoing headache. She had not previously taken any medication for the headache, and she had never taken any medication for headaches. Rather than start her on anything stronger, the physician suggested aspirin to see how she would react. Unfortunately the patient developed a rash after taking the aspirin and returned to see the physician who indicated she had suffered an adverse reaction to the aspirin. _____

25. A patient was seen in the emergency department for pain in his right arm after accidentally falling off his bicycle. The emergency department physician determined the patient had injured the arm as a result of the bicycle fall._____

# Infectious and Parasitic Diseases
## Codes 001–139

Codes in this chapter classify communicable infectious and parasitic diseases. Most categories describe a condition and the type of organism that causes it. For example, category 004, shigellosis, describes acute infectious dysentery caused by *Shigella* bacteria. This category's codes classify four groups of bacteria plus a code for other *specified Shigella* infections, which occur infrequently, and a code for *unspecified* shigellosis for use when the condition is insufficiently described in the medical documentation for specific code assignment.

---

### CODING TIP

*"Includes" Notes*

In the Tabular List, the word *includes* followed by descriptions of conditions helps the coder confirm the correct classification. These notes apply to the chapter, section, or category under which they appear. For example, the note *"Includes infection or food poisoning by Salmonella"* appears beneath category 003, Other salmonella infections, and applies to infection or food poisoning caused by any organism in the category—that is, all the codes that begin with 003.

---

### Provide the codes for the following diagnoses.

1. trichinosis _____

2. trichuriasis _____

3. Lyme disease _____

4. tabes dorsalis _____

5. ECHO virus _____

6. ovale malaria _____

7. Behçet's syndrome _____

8. primary genital syphilis _____

9. viral hepatitis A without mention of hepatic coma _____

10. rabies _____

11. tuberculous laryngitis, bacteriological examination not done _____

**For the following descriptions, check the "Include" note when assigning the code.**

12. chronic hepatitis E without mention of hepatic coma _____

13. Malta fever _____

14. amebic skin ulceration due to *Entamoeba histolytica* _____

15. chronic gonococcal cystitis _____

16. recurrent tick-borne fever _____

17. pertussis due to *Bordetella bronchiseptica* _____

18. gonococcal endometritis, three months' duration _____

19. intestinal infection due to *Campylobacter* _____

20. shingles _____

## Provide the diagnoses codes for the following case studies.

21. A patient who had been exposed to AIDS (acquired immune deficiency syndrome) in the past developed symptoms of the disease, was tested, and learned that the results were positive for AIDS.

    _____

22. For weeks a patient was ill with diarrhea and abdominal pain. After examination and blood tests were completed, it was determined the patient suffered from enteritis caused by the astrovirus.

    _____

23. A patient was suffering from a yeast infection of the skin and finger-nails. She made an appointment with her physician, and after examination and blood work, he determined that she suffered from candidal onychia.

    _____

24. After 3 weeks of fever and chest pain, a patient was seen by his physician who determined that something was wrong with the patient's pericardium, the outer lining of the heart. After laboratory workup and testing, it was determined the patient had Coxsackie pericarditis.

    _____

25. A young patient with strep throat went untreated for over 3 weeks and developed scarlatina anginosa.

    _____

# Neoplasms

## Codes 140–239

Codes in this chapter of the ICD-9-CM classify neoplasms, or tumors, which are growths that arise from normal tissue. Tumors are described according to their behavior as being one of four types: malignant (fast growing), benign (not spreading), of uncertain behavior (requiring further study), and of unspecified nature (insufficiently described for specific code assignment). Malignant tumors include primary, a tumor at the original site; secondary, a tumor that has spread, or *metastasized,* to another location from its primary site; and in situ, a noninvasive malignant tumor. Carcinoma in situ may also be referred to as *preinvasive cancer.*

In coding physicians' encounters with patients (physician coding), reporting suspected or possible conditions is avoided. Before pathology work identifies the behavior of a tumor, the condition can be classified with a code in the range 780–799 (Symptoms, Signs, or Ill-Defined Conditions), if applicable, or with V71.1 (observation for suspected malignant neoplasm, not found) or V76 (screening for malignant neoplasms).

---

### CODING TIP

*The Neoplasm Table*

The Alphabetic Index contains a Neoplasm Table that points to codes for neoplasms. The table lists the anatomical location in the first column. The next six columns classify the behavior of the neoplasm.

---

### Using the Neoplasm Table in the Alphabetic Index, assign codes to the following diagnoses.

1.  malignant primary neoplasm of the lower jawbone _____

2.  benign neoplasm of the pharynx _____

3.  neoplasm in situ, Wirsung's duct _____

4.  neoplastic growth on the skin of the hip, uncertain behavior _____

    _____

5.  secondary neoplasm on the posterior wall of the stomach _____

6.  unspecified neoplasm of the pericardium _____

7.  neoplasm of the mesopharynx, primary _____

8.  cancer in situ, distal esophagus _____

9. benign tumor of the midbrain _____

10. spinal column neoplasm, primary _____

## Using the Alphabetic Index and the Tabular List, provide codes for the following diagnoses.

11. subacute leukemia in remission _____

12. Hodgkin's granuloma, multiple lymph nodes _____

13. uterine fibromyoma _____

14. Letterer-Siwe disease, spleen _____

15. suspected primary carcinoma of the arm, screening test _____

16. ascites; possible carcinoma of the pancreas _____

17. cancer that has metastasized to the nose _____

18. cancer in situ of the temporal lobe _____

19. history of malignant neoplasm of stomach _____

20. screening mammogram, patient has family history of breast cancer and

    is considered high risk *(two codes)* _____

## Provide the diagnoses codes for the following case studies.

21. After noticing a smallish dark irregular spot on her lip, the patient was seen by her internist who biopsied the site. The pathology report came back as malignant melanoma. _____

22. While examining her patient during an annual physical, a physician noticed a nodule on the left shoulder. It was approximately 1 cm, and the physician was almost certain it was benign. She excised the nodule, and it was sent for pathology. The report indicated a dermatofibroma of the skin on the shoulder. _____

23. A patient with a history of abnormal pap smears is tested again. This time the result indicates a CINIII finding, or an in situ neoplasm of the cervix uteri. _____

24. This patient has a long history of respiratory infections, productive cough, and asthma. The physician has done recent testing to determine the cause of this extensive respiratory difficulty. The CT scan shows an anomaly, and the physician asks the patient to come in for another examination. His findings in the documentation indicate a neoplasm of the respiratory system. _____

25. Patient was in pain for several weeks in the sinus area. After ruling out sinusitis, the patient was referred to an otolaryngologist who examined the patient endoscopically and determined there was a lesion in the accessory sinuses. The lesion was biopsied, and the pathology report stated that the lesion was a carcinoma in situ of the accessory sinuses.

    _____

# Endocrine, Nutritional, and Metabolic Diseases, and Immunity Disorders

## Codes 240–279

Codes in this chapter of the ICD-9-CM classify a variety of conditions. The most common disease is diabetes mellitus, which may be either type I (the patient's health depends on receiving regular insulin injections and following a strict regimen to avoid serious complications) or type II (the patient's condition may be managed with medication, diet, and exercise, although a requirement for insulin may occur). Another common condition is obesity, in which body weight is beyond skeletal and physical requirements because of excessive accumulation of body fat. Obesity is associated with a number of primary conditions, such as coronary artery disease, gallbladder disease, high cholesterol, hypertension, and type II diabetes mellitus.

## CODING TIP

### *The Highest Level of Specificity— Fourth and Fifth Digits*

When a fifth-digit subclassification is provided, a five-digit code must be assigned. A four-digit code is used only when there is no five-digit code, and a three-digit code is assigned only when the category does not have four-digit codes. In other words, the coder should choose the most specific code available, selecting a four-digit code over a three-digit code and, likewise, choosing a five-digit code over a four-digit code. In the Tabular List of the ICD-9-CM, a mark (such as a check) is used to show a fifth-digit subclassification requirement. If a fifth digit is not required, do not add a zero or zeroes to a four-digit or three-digit code.

### Provide the codes for the following diagnoses.

1. congenital hypothyroidism _____

2. mucopolysaccharidosis _____

3. gouty arthropathy _____

4. macroglobulinemia _____

5. deficiency of vitamin K _____

6. medulloadrenal hyperfunction _____

7. kwashiorkor _____

8. Hashimoto's disease _____

9. Werner's syndrome _____

10. Lorain-Levi dwarfism _____

## Note the fifth-digit subclassification requirement when assigning codes for the following diagnoses.

11. Grave's disease _____

12. diabetes mellitus, type I, uncontrolled _____

13. diabetes mellitus, type II _____

14. diabetes with ketoacidosis, type II, controlled _____

15. insulin coma, patient with uncontrolled juvenile diabetes mellitus _____

16. diabetes with hypoglycemia, type I _____

17. uric acid nephrolithiasis _____

18. morbid obesity _____

19. Herrick's syndrome _____

20. obese patient encounter for dietary counseling (two codes) _____

## Provide diagnoses codes for the following case studies.

21. An adolescent boy has been seen annually by his internist who noticed a disturbing weight gain, some behavioral problems, and high blood sugar. Realizing the implication of this combination of problems could be based in the pituitary gland, the physician ordered tests and confirmed the diagnosis of Frohlich's syndrome. _____

22. Due to evidence of other metabolic disorders, a patient was asked to come in for urinalysis. The test results confirmed the physician's suspicion that amino acids were being excreted via the urine in abnormal amounts. The patient was diagnosed with cystinuria. _____

23. Patient presents with a 5-day history of excessive diarrhea and vomiting which has now resolved, but the patient is still unable to drink water or eat. The physician suspects gastroenteritis and schedules the patient for testing. At this point, however, the physician indicates a diagnosis of dehydration. _____

24. Treating a 60-year-old patient, the physician notices a swelling in the neck area and determines that the patient's thyroid is enlarged on one side. After blood work, which indicates increased levels of the thyroid hormone, the physician diagnosed a thyrocele. _____

25. A physician has been following a patient who recently arrived from a foreign country. As a result of his patient's depression, diarrhea, and unusual dermatitis, the physician orders lab work to determine what is the cause of his patient's symptoms. The result shows a niacin deficiency. On the basis of this finding, and the fact that the dermatitis is located only in body areas exposed to light, a diagnosis of pellagra is made.

_____

# Diseases of the Blood and Blood-Forming Organs

## Codes 280–289

Codes in this chapter of the ICD-9-CM classify diseases of the blood and blood-forming organs, such as anemia and coagulation defects.

---

### CODING TIP

#### The Colon and the Brace in the Tabular List

Two punctuation marks—the colon and the brace—are used in the Tabular List of the ICD-9-CM to introduce diagnostic terms that are connected to the term they follow. These modifying terms help the coder verify the correct code. For example, under subcategory 281.0 Pernicious anemia, the terms *Addison's, Biermer's,* and *congenital pernicious* each modify the term *anemia.*

---

### Provide the codes for the following diagnoses.

1. chlorotic anemia _____

2. anemia due to dietary deficiency of vitamin $B_{12}$ _____

3. sickle-cell anemia _____

4. hemophilia _____

5. hereditary hemolytic anemia _____

6. hereditary hemolytic anemia due to enzyme deficiency _____

7. stomatocytosis _____

8. specified hereditary hemolytic anemia

    not elsewhere classified _____

9. congenital elliptocytosis _____

10. iron deficiency anemia _____

11. Henoch's purpura _____

12. aplastic anemia due to chronic systemic disease _____

13. sideroblastic anemia _____

14. congenital dyserythropoietic anemia _____

15. Runeberg's disease _____

## Provide the codes for the diagnoses in these case studies.

16. After the birth of her first child, the patient bled profusely to the point of endangering her life. She mentioned to the obstetrician that her mother had had a similar problem when she was born. The lab results showed a deficiency in blood factor VII, indicative of von Willebrand's disease, which is congenital.

_____

_____

17. On several occasions, this patient noticed increased bleeding from even minor cuts or abrasions. Finally deciding to see her physician, the patient had lab work done, and the result indicated a low platelet count, with a diagnosis of thrombocytopenia.

_____

_____

18. After open heart surgery for blocked coronary arteries, the patient developed purplish spots on the leg that was used to harvest his vein for the graft material to be used in the heart bypass procedure. He had not injured the leg, but after years of smoking, his vascular system was compromised. After blood work was done, a diagnosis of secondary thrombocytopenia was given.

_____

_____

19. After years of untreated hypertension and development of end stage renal disease (ESRD), a patient also develops anemia. The physician explains that this is not an uncommon result of the ESRD and gives an additional diagnosis of anemia in end stage renal disease.

_____

_____

20. A patient with fatigue, shortness of breath, and weakness is seen. Lab work indicates a deficiency in the red blood cell membrane, and a diagnosis of congenital nonspherocytic anemia, type II is made.

_____

_____

NAME _____

# Mental Disorders

## Codes 290–319

Codes in this chapter of the ICD-9-CM classify the various types of mental disorders, including conditions of drug and alcohol dependency, Alzheimer's disease, schizophrenic disorders, and mood disturbances.

---

## CODING TIP

### The Abbreviations NEC and NOS

NEC and NOS have different meanings and uses. NEC stands for not elsewhere classified. This abbreviation appears with a term when there is no code that is specific for the condition. It means that no code matches the particular problem described in the diagnostic statement. In this case, the coder has specific documentation, but ICD-9-CM does not provide a code that matches the statement. NOS, which stands for not otherwise specified, means that the diagnostic statement does not provide enough information to classify the condition.

---

## Provide the codes for the following diagnoses.

1. mild mental retardation _____

2. depression _____

3. frontal lobe syndrome _____

4. tobacco dependence _____

5. subacute delirium _____

6. nonalcoholic Korsakoff's psychosis _____

7. neurotic anxiety disorder _____

8. depression with anxiety _____

9. panic attack _____

10. narcissistic personality disorder _____

## Note the fifth-digit subclassification requirement when assigning codes for the following diagnoses.

11. episodic cocaine abuse _____

12. active disintegrative psychosis _____

13. severe mixed manic-depressive psychosis _____

14. chronic catatonic type schizophrenic disorder _____

15. occasional amphetamine abuse _____

16. drunkenness _____

17. dependence on barbiturates and morphine _____

## Provide the diagnoses codes for the following case studies.

18. The patient presents with a 10-year history of drug abuse and is being seen today for evaluation of a 2-year history of continuous dependence on methadone.

    _____

    _____

19. Due to complaints from the school, a pediatrician is examining a 5-year-old child who is having mild tantrums so often that his parents are concerned that there is something physically wrong with him. The school feels the tantrums go beyond what is expected for the child's age. No physical explanation is found on examination.

    _____

    _____

20. A patient was brought to the emergency room after hours of rapid, excited speech, unexplained laughter, and constant, rapid movements. Friends were unable to determine why this was happening and were concerned. No drugs were found, and the physician decided this was a single episode of manic disorder and recommended the patient see his own physician the next day for a complete workup.

    _____

    _____

# Diseases of the Nervous System and Sense Organs
## Codes 320–389

Codes in this chapter of the ICD-9-CM classify diseases of the central nervous system, the peripheral nervous system, the eye, and the ear.

---

## CODING TIP

### "Code First Underlying Disease" Instruction

Some conditions require the assignment of two codes, one for the disease's etiology (origin or cause) and a second for its manifestation, or typical signs or symptoms. (On occasion, there is a single combination code for the etiology and the manifestation.) In the Alphabetic Index, a requirement for two codes is indicated when two codes appear after a term, the second of which is in brackets and italics. Likewise, the instruction "code first underlying disease" in the Tabular List indicates the need for two codes. (The alternative phrases "code first associated disorder" or "code first underlying disorder" may also be used.) The instruction appears below a code printed in italics. Codes shown in italics are never primary. These codes are for the *manifestation* only, not for the etiology, even when the diagnostic statement is written in that order.

---

**Provide the codes for the following diagnoses.**

1. Huntington's chorea _____

2. hereditary spastic paraplegia _____

3. paralysis _____

4. brachial plexus lesions _____

5. benign intracranial hypertension _____

6. blind hypotensive eye _____

7. cortical senile cataract _____

8. diplopia _____

9. visual field defect _____

10. achromatopsia _____

**Provide both the etiology and manifestation codes in the correct order. *Hint:*
Remember to check for fifth-digit subclassification requirements.**

11. toxic encephalitis due to exposure to mercury _____

12. childhood cerebral degeneration due to Hunter's disease _____

13. peripheral autonomic neuropathy in type II controlled diabetes _____

   _____

14. Eaton-Lambert syndrome due to pernicious anemia _____

15. myopathy from Addison's disease _____

16. retinal dystrophy in Fabry's disease _____

17. glaucoma in/with neurofibromatosis _____

18. diabetic cataract _____

19. exophthalmic ophthalmoplegia due to toxic diffuse goiter _____

20. chronic mycotic otitis externa because of otomycosis _____

## Provide the diagnoses codes for these case studies.

21. Patient presents today with difficulty in producing tears. After exami-
    nation the physician determined that the tear sac, or lacrimal sac, was
    narrowed. The diagnosis is stenosis of the lacrimal sac.

    _____

22. After suffering for 3 days with a fever and ear pain, the patient was seen
    by her physician. Upon examination the physician found purulent materi-
    al in the middle ear and diagnosed an acute case of serous otitis media.

    _____

23. A patient with both chronic and acute sinusitis comes in today because
    of a constant ringing in her right ear. Upon examination the physician
    determines that she has subjective tinnitus because the sound can only
    be heard by the patient.

    _____

24. After 2 days of discharge and redness in both eyes, a patient is seen by
    his internist. The internist determined the patient was suffering from
    conjunctivitis, specifically mucopurulent conjunctivitis.

    _____

25. Patient notices a halo around street lights and traffic lights when driv-
    ing at night. She has also noticed a lessening in her peripheral vision.
    Her ophthalmologist examines her eyes with the ophthalmoscope and
    does visual field testing. The results of these examinations indicate pri-
    mary open-angle glaucoma.

    _____

    _____

NAME _____

# Diseases of the Circulatory System
## Codes 390–459

Codes in this chapter of the ICD-9-CM classify a large group of circulatory system disorders. Many are complex, involving heart disease and serious vascular disorders.

---

### CODING TIP

*"Excludes" Notes*

In the Tabular List, the word *excludes* is followed by descriptions of conditions to help the coder confirm the correct classification. These notes apply to the chapter, section, or category under which they appear. For example, the note *"Excludes that with heart involvement"* appears beneath category 390, Rheumatic fever without mention of heart involvement. If a diagnostic statement mentions rheumatic arthritis, rheumatic fever, or articular rheumatism and heart involvement, this category is inappropriate.

---

### Provide the codes for the following diagnoses.

1. acute rheumatic endocarditis _____

2. chronic rheumatic pericarditis _____

3. angina pectoris _____

4. preinfarction angina _____

5. chronic myocardial ischemia _____

6. chronic primary pulmonary hypertension _____

7. acute endocarditis _____

8. constrictive pericarditis _____

9. aortic valve stenosis _____

10. cardiomegaly _____

11. heart failure following cardiac surgery _____

12. meningococcal infective endocarditis _____

13. Spens' syndrome _____

**Be alert for fifth-digit subclassification requirements when assigning codes for the following diagnoses.**

14. acute myocardial infarction _____

15. initial care of acute myocardial infarction of anterolateral wall _____

16. occlusion of basilar artery with cerebral infarction _____

17. cerebral thrombosis _____

18. stenosis of vertebral artery _____

19. Beck's syndrome _____

20. sinus tachycardia _____

**Provide codes for the diagnoses in these case studies.**

21. A 70-year-old man has been experiencing shortness of breath and fatigue. His internist referred him to a cardiologist who performed a stress test that was abnormal. An echocardiogram indicated a problem on the right side of the heart. A cardiac catheterization was performed, and it was determined that the patient suffered from an obstruction in the tricuspid valve between the right atrium and the right ventricle.

_____

22. Three years ago this patient suffered an acute myocardial infarction. He has been treated with medication, exercise, and diet; after 8 weeks his condition was no longer considered acute. He comes in today for his 3-year follow-up visit, and he is completely without any symptoms. His diagnosis is healed (old) myocardial infarction.

_____

23. A patient has been complaining of chest pain, but his EKGs and a stress test are normal. An echocardiogram is performed showing layers of the pericardium had adhered to each other. Diagnosis: Soldier's patches.

_____

24. A patient with long-term liver disease has his blood work checked. Lab results indicate a low hematocrit, and his physician suspects internal bleeding. An esophagoscopy is done showing that the patient has bleeding esophageal varicose veins.

_____

25. A patient calls his internist. He feels like he is suffocating and he has chest pain. It started when he was running with his grandchildren. He noticed a similar reaction after cutting the lawn recently. After examination, EKG, and an attempted stress test, the physician diagnosed stenocardia.

_____

# Diseases of the Circulatory System *continued*

## CODING TIP

### *Hypertension*

Hypertension is a diagnosis related to high blood pressure. Almost all cases are due to unknown causes. This is called essential hypertension and is the primary diagnosis. In the few cases where the cause is known, the hypertension is called secondary, and its code is listed after the code for the cause.

Within the essential hypertension category, there are three subcategories: *malignant* (401.0), *benign* (401.1), and *unspecified* (401.9). Malignant hypertension is an extremely serious condition, so it is always documented as malignant. Benign hypertension is a relatively mild and often chronic condition. If the diagnostic statement does not contain either word, the hypertension is coded as unspecified. Hypertension can affect the heart and/or the kidneys. Hypertensive heart disease and hypertensive renal disease are coded under the categories 402 to 404.

Note that a diagnosis of hypertension is different from "high (or elevated) blood pressure." If the diagnosis does not include *hypertension,* the statement is coded 796.2, elevated blood pressure reading without diagnosis of hypertension.

The Alphabetic Index contains a detailed table to point to the various types of hypertensive disease, including its effect on pregnancy. Hypertension is often indicated as a coexisting condition with other conditions. When these diagnoses appear, two codes must be assigned, one for the first condition and one for the hypertension, which is secondary in this case.

**Using the Hypertension Table in the Alphabetic Index, assign codes to the following diagnoses.**

26. benign hypertension due to brain tumor _____

27. unspecified hypertension due to renal artery stenosis _____

28. secondary malignant hypertension due to Cushing's disease

_____

29 accelerated hypertension _____

30. intermittent vascular hypertensive disease _____

Following the normal procedure, provide the codes for the following diagnoses. Some diagnoses require two codes.

31. rheumatic aortic insufficiency and congestive heart failure _____

32. mitral and aortic valve insufficiency and atrial flutter _____

33. acute pericarditis caused by uremia _____

34. heart failure due to benign hypertension _____

35. hypertrophy of the heart due to malignant hypertension _____

36. cardiomyopathy due to excessive alcohol consumption _____

37. angina decubitus and essential hypertension _____

38. tuberculosis (unspecified) and endocarditis _____

39. peripheral angiopathy due to diabetes mellitus _____

40. inflamed varicose veins on the leg _____

# Diseases of the Respiratory System

## Codes 460–519

Codes in this chapter of the ICD-9-CM classify respiratory illnesses such as pneumonia, chronic obstructive pulmonary disease, and asthma.

---

### CODING TIP

#### *Chronic versus Acute Conditions*

Acute conditions—those with relatively sudden or severe problems—are reported with the specific code that is designated acute, if provided in the ICD-9-CM. Chronic conditions—those that continue over a long period of time or recur frequently—are reported each time the patient receives care for that condition. Some encounters cover treatment for both an acute and a chronic condition. If both an acute illness and a chronic condition are treated in an encounter and each has a code, list the acute code first. In some cases, a single code covers both types of the condition, so only one code is reported.

---

### Provide the codes for the following diagnoses.

1. bronchiectasis without acute exacerbation _____

2. adenoid vegetations _____

3. deviated nasal septum _____

4. cellulitis of vocal cords _____

5. nasopharyngeal polyp _____

6. peritonsillar abscess _____

7. asbestosis _____

8. lung abscess _____

9. allergic bronchopulmonary aspergillosis _____

10. influenza due to identified novel H1N1 (swine flu) _____

## Some of the following diagnoses require two codes.

11. pneumonia in cytomegalic inclusion disease _____

12. pneumonia due to *Pseudomonas* _____

13. acute and chronic respiratory failure _____

14. adenoviral pneumonia and allergic bronchitis _____

15. asthma with chronic obstructive pulmonary disease _____

16. acute bronchitis with chronic obstructive pulmonary disease _____

17. acute pulmonary manifestations due to radiation _____

18. hypertrophy of nasal turbinates _____

19. hyperplasia of tonsils with adenoids _____

20. acute bronchiolitis due to RSV _____

## Provide codes for these case studies.

21. After moving to South Carolina, a patient noticed increasing shortness of breath and wheezing, and was diagnosed with asthma. This morning she presents with greater difficulty in breathing and her wheezing has become much worse—it had started suddenly during the night.

_____

22. A 12-year-old boy starts complaining of itchy eyes, runny nose, sneezing; he says he feel stuffy. His problem seems to coincide with the trees and flowers starting to bloom. His pediatrician diagnosed allergic rhinitis from exposure to pollen.

_____

23. The patient presents with a 2-year history of a productive cough with unknown etiology, which is now more severe. The physician documents a diagnosis of acute and chronic obstructive bronchitis.

_____

24. After 2 weeks of throat pain, the patient realized that he also was running a fever. After dealing with the fever for 3 days, he sees his physician, who indicates a diagnosis of acute infective tonsillitis.

_____

25. A 32-year-old patient with virtually a lifetime history of allergies has been seeing her physician almost five times a year for pain in the area behind her cheekbones and purulent nasal discharge. The physician documents that the patient has chronic maxillary sinus infections.

_____

# Diseases of the Digestive System
## Codes 520–579

Codes in this chapter of the ICD-9-CM classify diseases of the digestive system. Codes are listed according to anatomical location, beginning with the oral cavity and continuing through the intestines.

---

### CODING TIP

*Combination Codes*

Some conditions in the ICD-9-CM are classified with combination codes that cover both the illness, such as gastric or peptic ulcers, and a commonly associated condition, such as hemorrhage (bleeding) and/or perforation. Check carefully during the coding process to verify whether a combination code classifies both the etiology and the manifestation of the documented diagnosis.

---

**Provide the codes for the following diagnoses.**

1. anal abscess _____

2. appendicitis _____

3. reflux esophagitis _____

4. alveolitis of the jaw _____

5. plaque induced acute gingivitis _____

6. arthralgia of temporomandibular joint _____

7. anodontia _____

8. glossodynia _____

9. sialoadenitis _____

10. perforated esophagus _____

11. segmental ileitis _____

12. fecal impaction _____

13. cholestatic cirrhosis _____

### Some of the following diagnoses require two codes.

14. hepatitis in mumps _____

15. hepatitis in Coxsackie virus disease _____

16. gastrojejunal ulcer with obstruction, hemorrhage, and perforation

    _____

17. strawberry gallbladder _____

18. acute and chronic cholecystitis _____

19. recurrent bilateral inguinal hernia _____

20. liver damage because of chronic alcoholism _____

### Provide codes for the diagnoses in these case studies.

21. Patient complains of difficulty swallowing with an almost constant
    burning sensation in the lower chest area. An x-ray is performed with
    fluoroscopy. The x-ray shows a protrusion/hernia of the stomach
    through the opening of the esophagus where it joins the stomach
    (esophageal hiatus).

    _____

22. Two months after surgery for a partial colectomy, the patient comes in
    to see his surgeon for ongoing abdominal pain. Upon examination, the
    surgeon finds adhesions in the patient's peritoneum.

    _____

23. A dialysis patient who recently changed over to continual ambulatory
    peritoneal dialysis complains of abdominal pain. The physician deter-
    mines that the patient has peritonitis.

    _____

24. A patient has been suffering with stomach pain, cramps, and diarrhea for
    2 months; her weight is dropping dramatically. The physician orders a
    CT scan, and the findings indicate Crohn's disease.

    _____

25. Patient has suffered for years with stomach pain and now sees his
    physician because he has started vomiting. In the course of their dis-
    cussion the patient mentions that he gets some relief from drinking
    milk. The physician schedules an endoscopy and finds a perforated
    peptic ulcer.

    _____

    _____

# Diseases of the Genitourinary System

## Codes 580–629

Codes in this chapter of the ICD-9-CM classify diseases of the male and female genitourinary (GU) systems, such as infections of the genital tract, renal disease, conditions of the prostate, and problems with the cervix, vulva, and breast.

---

### CODING TIP

#### "Use Additional Code" Instruction

If a code is followed in the Tabular List by the instruction "use additional code" or "code also" (or another phrase meaning the same thing), two codes are required. In some cases, the additional code classifies an associated condition or organism. If the underlying disease must be coded first, the instruction is "Code first" . . . , and code order is the same as shown in the Alphabetic Index—etiology followed by manifestation.

---

**Provide the codes for the following diagnoses.**

1. renal failure _____

2. ureteric stone _____

3. mobile kidney _____

4. chronic interstitial cystitis _____

5. abscess of urethral gland _____

6. male infertility _____

7. galactocele _____

8. acute salpingitis and oophoritis _____

9. uterine endometriosis _____

10. ovarian cyst _____

**Provide two codes for each of the following diagnostic statements. Remember to check for fifth-digit subclassification requirements and to list codes in the correct order, if it is specified.**

11. uremic pericarditis _____

12. enlarged prostate with urge and stress incontinence _____

13. prostatitis in blastomycosis _____

14. vaginitis due to *Staphylococcus* _____

15. female infertility due to postoperative peritubal adhesions

    _____

16. acute cystitis due to *Escherichia coli* organism _____

17. nephritis due to diabetes mellitus _____

18. pyelonenephritis due to renal tuberculosis _____

19. acute prostatitis due to *Streptococcus* _____

20. vulvovaginal gland abscess and female stress incontinence

    _____

## Provide codes for the following case studies.

21. The patient is seen for her annual gynecological exam, and a pap smear is taken. The results show a mild dysplasia of the cervix. _____

22. A 30-year-old woman has recently started doing her own breast exams and notices a bumpy consistency to her breasts, with some mild pain, particularly just before and after her menstrual period. Due to her concern, she sees her gynecologist who after examining her documents a diagnosis of fibrocystic breast disease._____

23. A 58-year-old woman sees her gynecologist because she is having urinary problems. She complains that when she sneezes or coughs, she urinates involuntarily, even though she has recently emptied her bladder. It even occurs when she tries to lift one of her grandchildren. The physician diagnoses stress incontinence._____

24. A patient with a 6-year history of adult onset diabetes is seen for follow up of her diabetic condition. The physician does lab work and weighs the patient who shows a considerable weight gain and edema. The lab work results indicate a large amount of protein in the urine. The physician documents nephrosis. _____

25. Patient presents with vaginal bleeding and pain. After the physical exam, the gynecologist recommends a diagnostic laparoscopy based on her findings. During the laparoscopy, the gynecologist finds a chocolate cyst in the ovary. _____

# Complications of Pregnancy, Childbirth, and the Puerperium
## Codes 630–679

Codes in this chapter of the ICD-9-CM classify conditions that are involved with pregnancy, childbirth, and the puerperium. Many categories require a fifth-digit subclassification based on when the complications occur (referred to as the episode of care), either before birth (antepartum), during, or after birth (postpartum). Valid fifth digits are usually shown in brackets next to the subcategory.

---

### CODING TIP

*Mothers' Conditions*

Codes in this chapter (Chapter 11) of ICD-9-CM are assigned to conditions of the mother only, not of the infant. They cover the course of pregnancy and childbirth from conception through the puerperium, which is the 6-week period following delivery. Codes for conditions that affect newborns are in ICD-9-CM's Chapter 15.

---

### Provide codes for the following diagnoses.

1. hydatidiform mole _____

2. abdominal pregnancy without intrauterine pregnancy _____

3. complete spontaneous abortion complicated by renal failure _____

4. incomplete spontaneous abortion with complications _____

5. legally induced abortion _____

6. complete abortion complicated by shock _____

7. abortion _____

8. hemorrhage in early pregnancy _____

9. premature separation of placenta _____

10. mild hyperemesis gravidarum _____

11. Rh incompatibility _____

12. delivery complicated by short umbilical cord _____

13. puerperal pulmonary embolism _____

14. nipple fissure in fourth week after childbirth _____

15. delivery complicated by inverted uterus _____

16. postpartum fibrinolysis _____

**Provide two codes for each of the following diagnostic statements. Remember to check for fifth-digit subclassification requirements and to list codes in the correct order, if it is specified.**

17. normal delivery of single liveborn _____

18. normal delivery of liveborn twins _____

19. normal delivery of quadruplets, three liveborn and one stillborn

_____

20. delivery complicated by obstructed labor caused by face presentation

_____

**Provide codes for the following case studies.**

21. A pregnant patient finds herself bleeding and is unable to staunch the bleeding. She goes to the emergency department where the physician informs the patient that she is hemorrhaging.

_____

22. The patient is frazzled to find herself still pregnant after 41 weeks. She had planned to deliver after the "normal" 39 weeks and is having difficulty adjusting to this delay.

_____

23. This 30-year-old is seeing her obstetrician during her first pregnancy for regular follow-up care during her 25th week of pregnancy. She mentions the swelling in her legs and unusual fatigue. The physician does a blood workup which reveals an abnormal blood glucose. He reassures his patient that she does not have diabetes, but what is referred to as gestational diabetes, and he fully expects her blood glucose to return to normal after the baby is delivered.

_____

24. A day after delivering her baby, the patient finds herself in additional discomfort and discovers a swollen area on her vulva. The obstetrician comes in to examine her and finds she has a hematoma.

_____

25. During the eighth month of her pregnancy, the patient contacts her obstetrician because of the discomfort from the baby's position. She is also experiencing a swollen, reddened area on her calf that is painful. The obstetrician has her come in immediately and finds she has a deep vein thrombosis on the left leg. The patient is informed she must get off her feet and lie with the leg elevated, using warm compresses.

_____

# Diseases of the Skin and Subcutaneous Tissue

## Codes 680–709

Codes in this chapter of the ICD-9-CM classify skin infections, inflammations, and other diseases.

---

### CODING TIP

#### *Notes at the Beginning of a Chapter*

Coders should be aware that an entire chapter or section may be subject to "Excludes" or "Includes" notes, based on the note's location. For example, the first section in this chapter (680–686) begins with a note excluding certain skin infections that are classified in Chapter 1.

---

### Provide codes for the following diagnoses.

1. allergic urticaria _____

2. sebaceous cyst _____

3. hirsutism _____

4. ingrowing nail _____

5. acquired keratoderma _____

6. clavus _____

7. lichenification _____

8. parapsoriasis _____

9. Ritter's disease _____

10. dermatosis herpetiformis _____

11. DSAP (disseminated superficial actinic porokeratosis) _____

12. herald patch _____

13. paronychia of big toe _____

14. psoriatic arthropathy _____

**Provide two codes for each of the following diagnostic statements. Remember to check for fifth-digit subclassification requirements and to list codes in the correct order, if it is specified.**

15. winter itch and prurigo nodularis _____

16. photoallergic response due to uric acid metabolism drug _____

17. abscess of cheek due to *Staphylococcus aureus* _____

18. seborrhea and pustular acne _____

19. prickly heat rash and hidradenitis suppurative _____

20. boils on wrist and shoulder _____

## Provide codes for the following case studies.

21. A teenage patient volunteers to help out at the local homeless shelter. She offers to do dishes there every day after school. After two weeks, she realizes that the rash she has developed is not going away, and she sees her doctor who recognizes that she has contact dermatitis caused by the dish detergent.

   _____

   _____

22. An active, healthy 50-year-old patient is distressed to find several groups of skin eruptions on her lower abdomen and under her arms. Her internist sends her to a dermatologist who diagnoses Sneddon-Wilkinson syndrome.

   _____

   _____

23. A patient noticed a hardened area of skin on her forearm that appears to have some thickness to it. She sees a dermatologist who documents that she has a localized dermatosis.

   _____

   _____

24. An elderly man is hospitalized and subsequently placed on a ventilator. Due to his condition he is unable to move on his own or to be moved. As a result, he develops a stage 1 decubitus ulcer on his lower back.

   _____

   _____

25. A young patient is plagued with blackheads, and his PCP sends him to a dermatologist who provides treatment and documents that the patient has a form of acne known as comedo.

   _____

   _____

# Diseases of the Musculoskeletal System and Connective Tissue

## Codes 710–739

Codes in this chapter of the ICD-9-CM classify conditions of the bones and joints—arthropathies (joint disorders), dorsopathies (back disorders), rheumatism, and other diseases.

### CODING TIP

#### Fifth-Digit Subclassifications by Site

This chapter (Chapter 13) opens with a description of the fifth digits to be used for many categories. The subclassifications are organized by body site, from unspecified to multiple. The list also identifies the bones and joints that are included in each fifth digit. Remember to refer to this master list, because later in the chapter this subclassification appears in shortened form before the category and in brackets next to the code and description.

### Provide the codes for the following diseases.

1. hallux varus, right great toe _____

2. senile osteoporosis _____

3. bunion _____

4. limb pain _____

5. pain in lower back _____

6. cervicalgia _____

7. Schmorl's nodes of the lumbar region _____

8. calcaneal spur _____

9. patellar chondromalacia _____

10. systemic sclerosis _____

11. old rupture of meniscus of scapula _____

12. metatarsal arthralgia _____

13. Paget's bone disease _____

14. aseptic necrosis of medial femoral condyle _____

15. Legg-Calvé-Perthes disease _____

**Provide two codes for each of the following diagnostic statements. Remember to check for fourth- and fifth-digit requirements and to list codes in the correct order, if it is specified.**

16. upper arm arthropathy in Behçet's syndrome _____

17. arthropathic knee associated with ulcerative enterocolitis _____

18. vertebral column osteopathy due to infantile paralytic poliomyelitis

   _____

19. chronic osteomyelitis of glenohumeral joint and elbow joint

   _____

20. ruptured extensor and flexor tendons, hand _____

**Provide codes for the following case studies.**

21. The patient complains of pain in the lower leg. No injury has occurred, and the patient is otherwise healthy. A CT scan reveals osteomyelitis of the lower leg, and her physician further specifies her condition as acute.

   _____

22. A patient with long-term rheumatoid arthritis develops knee pain extending into the lower leg. X-rays are taken, and the radiologist finds a synovial cyst in the popliteal space of the knee, commonly known as Baker's cyst.

   _____

23. Five months ago, the patient suffered an ankle fracture. He is still in pain and feels that "something's not right." X-rays are taken of the original fracture site, and the findings are that the ankle has healed in misalignment—a malunion.

   _____

24. A 7-year-old boy is brought to the doctor because his left foot has turned inward and the heel has raised up. The problem may be a result of the boy's cerebral palsy, but this problem would have appeared earlier. For now the physician indicates he has acquired club foot of the left leg.

   _____

25. A 12-year-old's parents notice that their daughter is walking differently and appears to favor one side. They bring her the pediatrician who finds that the patient has a sideward curvature of the spine in the T1–T12 area, or thoracogenic scoliosis.

   _____

# Congenital Anomalies

## Codes 740–759

Codes in this brief ICD-9-CM chapter classify anomalies, malformations, and diseases that exist at birth. Unlike acquired disorders, congenital conditions are either hereditary or due to influencing factors during gestation.

---

### CODING TIP

*Congenital Anomalies and Patients' Ages*

Although congenital anomalies are defined as existing at birth, they do not always immediately affect the patient. As examples, normal human beings have 33 vertebrae, but a person without the normal number may be asymptomatic, and patients with dominant polycystic disease may not experience impaired function until adulthood. The classifications for congenital anomalies thus are not related to patients' ages.

---

### Provide codes for the following diagnoses.

1. congenital absence of vertebra _____

2. unilateral congenital hip dislocation _____

3. exstrophy of urinary bladder _____

4. undescended testis _____

5. congenital cystic liver disease _____

6. Hirschsprung's disease _____

7. aglossia _____

8. web of larynx _____

9. scimitar syndrome _____

10. posterior atresia of nares _____

11. cleft palate with cleft lip _____

12. pancreatic hypoplasia _____

13. autosomal dominant polycystic kidney _____

14. multiple symphalangy _____

15. deformity of clavicle, congenital _____

16. translocation Down's syndrome _____

17. hereditary trophedema _____

## Provide codes for the following case studies.

18. A newborn has difficulty breathing almost immediately after birth. The pediatrician's examination shows that the larynx is narrowed, almost completely stenosed, and an alternative airway needs to be created immediately.

   _____

   _____

19. A newborn shows difficulty with urination. The examination reveals that the urethra has failed to develop (atresia).

   _____

   _____

20. Shortly after a baby's birth, the pediatrician finds a dilated bladder and ureters and the absence of the lower rectus abdominis muscle, also known as prune belly syndrome.

   _____

   _____

# Certain Conditions Originating in the Perinatal Period

## Codes 760–779

Codes in this chapter of the ICD-9-CM classify conditions of the fetus or the newborn infant, the neonate, up to 28 days after birth.

---

### CODING TIP

#### *Infants' Conditions*

Codes in this chapter of the ICD-9-CM (Chapter 15) are assigned only to conditions of the infant, not of the mother. (Codes for conditions that affect the management of the mother's pregnancy are in Chapter 11.) They cover the perinatal period, which is the period from shortly before birth until 28 days following delivery. When the hospitalization that results in the birth is to be coded, these codes are secondary to codes from categories V30 through V39. Note the use of the fourth digit to designate the birth location and of the fifth digit to specify hospital births.

---

### Provide codes for the following diagnoses.

1. prematurity _____

2. fetal alcohol syndrome _____

3. fetus affected by the mother's malnutrition _____

4. neonatal hepatitis _____

5. respiratory distress syndrome _____

6. hyperthermia in newborn _____

7. anemia of prematurity _____

8. convulsions in newborn _____

9. neonatal superficial hematoma _____

10. congenital rubella _____

11. neonatal *Candida* infection _____

12. moderate birth asphyxia _____

## Provide a V code and a code from the range 760–779 for the following diagnoses.

13. hospital birth of living child, infant is premature and weighs 2000 grams

   _____

14. hospital birth of twin, mate liveborn, neonatal pulmonary immaturity

   _____

15. full-term birth in hospital of living male child, delivered by cesarean section, with neonatal transient hyperthyroidism

   _____

16. postterm birth in hospital of twin, mate stillborn

   _____

17. premature birth of female twins, first child delivered in ambulance en route to hospital, second child delivered in hospital

   _____

## Provide codes for the following case studies.

18. Shortly after birth, the newborn was taking quick breaths, indicating shallow breathing, with some evidence of cyanosis. After her examination, the pediatrician reassured the parents it was a transitory problem that would resolve on its own in about three days, but they would give the baby some oxygen in the meantime—the condition is often referred to as wet lung syndrome.

   _____

   _____

19. A pediatrician became concerned when he noticed that the newborn was somewhat jaundiced and had an enlarged spleen. Laboratory studies showed that the newborn suffered from anemia caused by RH isoimmunization.

   _____

   _____

20. Shortly before her labor started, a patient became short of breath and had difficulty walking. Her examination at the hospital showed an excess of amniotic fluid or hydramnios, which would account for her symptoms.

   _____

   _____

# Symptoms, Signs, and Ill-Defined Conditions
## Codes 780–799

Codes in this chapter of the ICD-9-CM classify patients' signs, symptoms, and ill-defined conditions for which a definitive diagnosis cannot be made. In physician coding, these codes are always used instead of coding "rule out," "probable," or "suspected" conditions.

## CODING TIPS

### High Blood Pressure

High (or elevated) blood pressure is classified to code 796.2, "elevated blood pressure reading without diagnosis of hypertension." This diagnosis is not the same as hypertension. (Compare this condition with that described in the Coding Tip on page 23.)

### HIV Codes

HIV coding is complex. When a diagnosis of HIV infection has been made, code 042 is used to classify any of the many terms used for this condition, such as AIDS (acquired immunodeficiency syndrome) and HIV disease. When a patient with no related symptoms has a screening test for HIV infection, code V73.89 is used. If the test results are positive for HIV infection but the patient shows no symptoms, code V08 is used. If, however, the test result is reported as "nonspecific serologic evidence of HIV," code 795.71 is used.

## Provide codes for the following diagnoses.

1. coma _____

2. fainting _____

3. abnormal electrocardiogram _____

4. viremia _____

5. abnormal blood glucose tolerance test _____

6. splenomegaly _____

7. urge incontinence _____

8. wheezing _____

9. hiccough _____

10. fever _____

11. ascites in the lower left quadrant of the abdomen _____

12. mass in epigastric area of abdomen _____

13. exanthem _____

14. nausea with vomiting _____

15. nosebleed _____

## Provide two codes for each of the following diagnostic statements. Remember to check for fourth- and fifth-digit requirements and to list codes in the correct order, if it is specified.

16. elevated blood pressure and nervousness _____

17. pallor and flushing _____

18. gangrene due to diabetes _____

19. continuous urinary incontinence because of complete uterovaginal

    prolapse _____

20. precordial pain and hyperventilation _____

## Provide codes for the following case studies.

21. A patient's wife goes to the doctor with her husband. She is concerned about his excessive, deep sleep. Often, she is unable to wake him. She also mentions that her husband will stop breathing during these episodes and she lies awake waiting for him to start again. The patient is sent for sleep studies which show that he suffers from hypersomnia and sleep apnea. _____

22. A young woman sees her internist. She is very concerned about her lack of energy, constant fatigue, and headache. She also has a chronic sore throat, and, at times, her lymph nodes are swollen. At the present time she does not have a fever, but periodically that is also a symptom. Many tests are done, none completely are definitive, and the internist documents chronic fatigue syndrome. _____

23. A man comes in to the emergency department in excruciating pain. At this point he is not sure he can determine the origin of the pain, but it seems to be located in the back, high up on the right side. He is almost unable to walk and states the pain is worse than having a fractured bone. The ED physician suspects kidney stones, but until tests are done he documents renal colic. _____

24. A 30-year-old woman starts to notice that she can feel her heart beat in her chest. She is healthy, exercises, and cannot correlate these episodes with any activity or occurrence. She is seen by her physician who will set her up for laboratory studies and cardiac studies. Until he has those findings, he indicates a diagnosis of palpitations. _____

25. Patient has been exposed to HIV, is not symptomatic of the illness, but wants to be tested for the disease. His blood (serology) test comes back as nonspecific. _____

# Injury and Poisoning
## Codes 800–999

Codes in this chapter of the ICD-9-CM classify injuries and wounds such as fractures, dislocations, sprains, strains, internal injuries, and traumatic injuries. The chapter also includes a section covering poisoning and a section for the late effects of injuries and poisoning. Often, E codes are also used to identify the cause of the injury or poisoning.

## CODING TIPS

### Open versus Closed Fractures

Classifications of fractures in ICD-9-CM carry a fourth digit based on whether they are open or closed. In a closed fracture, the broken bone does not pierce the skin. An open fracture involves a break through the skin. If the fracture is not indicated as open or closed, code it as closed. A fifth digit is often required for the specific anatomical site.

### Burns

Code burns with two codes: the first code for the burn's severity/body site, and the second code for its extent, known as total body surface area (TBSA):

1. Severity/site codes are grouped by sections of the body. Severity is one of three degrees: first-degree, in which the epidermis is damaged; second-degree, in which both the epidermis and the dermis are damaged; and third-degree, in which all three layers of the skin are damaged. Assign a fifth digit to further specify the site of the burn.

2. An additional code from the category 948 describes the TBSA involved based on the rule of nines (head and neck, 9%; each arm, 9%; each leg, 18%; front of trunk, 18%; back of trunk, 18%; perineum, 1%). The fourth digit shows the percentage of body surface (TBSA) for all burns. Use a fifth digit to classify the percentage of TBSA affected by third-degree burns; if it is none or less than 10%, use the fifth digit 0. Study the illustration at the top of page 44.

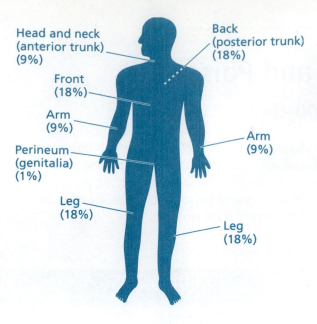

Head and neck
(anterior trunk)
(9%)

Back
(posterior trunk)
(18%)

Front
(18%)

Arm
(9%)

Arm
(9%)

Perineum
(genitalia)
(1%)

Leg
(18%)

Leg
(18%)

## Provide codes for the following diagnoses.

1. open fracture of nasal bones _____

2. closed fracture of sacrum and coccyx _____

3. open fracture of lumbar with spinal cord injury _____

4. closed fracture of big toe _____

5. metacarpophalangeal joint sprain _____

6. strained sacroiliac ligament _____

7. concussion with moderate loss of consciousness _____

8. internal laceration to lung with open wound into thorax _____

9. ocular laceration _____

10. open wound of nasal septum _____

11. complicated wound of upper arm _____

12. black eye _____

13. injury to auditory nerve _____

14. immediate shock after an injury _____

15. animal bite on knee _____

16. rupture of rotator cuff (traumatic) _____

17. closed posterior humeral dislocation _____

18. closed Dupuytren's fracture _____

19. closed fracture of the acromial process _____

# Injury and Poisoning *continued*

20. greenstick fracture, condylar process, mandible _____

21. open fracture of base of skull, with cerebral laceration, contusion, and

    concussion _____

22. ruptured superior vena cava _____

23. closed fracture of cervical vertebra with spinal nerve injury, C1–C4 ____

24. fracture of distal phalanges _____

25. pneumohemothorax _____

## Provide codes for these case studies.

26. Patient went to the emergency department after a fall in his home. He
    tripped on a rug, and when he fell, the front of his neck hit the arm of
    his sofa. The area is very sore, and he is concerned that he may have
    further complications. He is examined, and the ED physician docu-
    ments esophageal bruise. _____

27. A teenager practicing magic tricks is taken to the emergency room
    because he swallowed a nickel. The ED physician suggested he wait for
    nature to take its course. If that is not successful, he should see his
    own doctor at a later time. _____

28. After falling off his skateboard, the patient noticed a large bruise on his
    heel that looked like it was filled with blood. The physician diagnosed
    a hematoma on his heel as a result of his skateboard injury. _____

29. Patient presents with a portion of his left ear torn away after a motorcy-
    cle accident. The physician diagnosed left ear avulsion. _____

30. A 10-year-old girl comes to the ED. Her wrist is at an unusual angle,
    and she is in great pain. She was learning to skate for the first time and
    fell, using her hand to block her fall. X-rays are taken and the findings
    are that she has a fractured wrist _____

## Provide an injury code and an E code for each of the following diagnostic statements.

31. 7 ribs fractured due to fall from forklift truck _____

32. lacerations to hand from broken glass _____

33. forearm crushed under packing crate _____

34. bruise on buttock from fall during a horseback ride _____

35. snowblower accident caused multiple open wounds of lower limb

    _____

**Provide two codes for each of the following burns.**

36. third-degree burns of face, head, and neck (*Hint:* Provide a code for the burn degree and location, and a code for the 9% TBSA third-degree burn.) _____

_____

37. first-degree burn of thigh, lower leg, and foot _____

38. blistered palms _____

39. full-thickness skin loss of front and back of trunk _____

40. third-degree burns of both legs and back _____

---

## CODING TIP

### *Poisoning versus Adverse Effects*

Poisoning refers to the medical result of the incorrect use of a substance. This is different from accidental harm caused by a reaction to the correct dosage of a drug, called adverse effects. The Table of Drugs and Chemicals following the Alphabetic Index lists these agents alphabetically, and Column 1 contains the code for the poisoning. Use the table first to point to a code that you verify in the Tabular List under categories 960–979.

---

**Identify the codes for the following substances in the Table of Drugs and Chemicals.**

41. carbitol _____

42. calomel _____

43. iron compounds _____

44. soluble hexobarbitone _____

45. hornet sting _____

**Provide codes for the following diagnoses.**

46. tick paralysis _____

47. ampicillin taken in error _____

48. overdose of levodopa _____

49. toxic effect of petroleum products _____

50. Minamata disease _____

51. toxic effect of rubbing alcohol _____

# Injury and Poisoning *continued*

52. toxic effect, fumes of lead salts _____

53. heat cramps _____

54. accidental hypothermia _____

55. heat prostration _____

56. toxic effect of lye _____

57. poisoning by topical dental drugs _____

58. poisoning from local anesthetic _____

59. poisoning by psychotropic agent _____

60. methadone poisoning _____

61. overdose of ovarian hormones _____

62. poisoning by coronary vasodilator _____

63. coumarin poisoning _____

64. radiation sickness _____

65. anaphylactic shock after eating peanuts _____

## CODING TIP

### Late Effects

A late, or residual, effect is a condition that remains after an acute illness or injury. It may occur soon after the acute phase or later in life. Late effects are indicated by expressions such as "late," "due to an old . . ." or "due to a previous . . ." followed by the cause. Check late effects in the Alphabetic Index for the location of the applicable code. Two codes are required. Code the specific residual (late) effect first; then list the code for its cause.

## For the following late effects of injuries, provide two codes in the correct order.

66. nausea as a late effect of radiation sickness _____

67. pain from an old fractured shoulder blade _____

68. swelling due to old contusion of knee _____

69. abdominal mass due to a previous spleen injury _____

70. abnormal posture due to old sciatic nerve injury _____

# Coding Quiz: ICD-9-CM

NAME _____

_____ 1. Select the correct code for a personal history of cervical cancer.

&#9312; V16.41
&#9313; 180.9
&#9314; V10.41
&#9315; V10.40

_____ 2. Which is the correct code for a liveborn infant delivered by cesarean delivery in the hospital?

&#9312; V27.0
&#9313; V30.01
&#9314; V30
&#9315; V43.6

_____ 3. Select the correct code(s) for a patient who suffered an open fracture of the left radius in a fall from a moped on a highway.

&#9312; 813.05
&#9313; 813.91, E818.2
&#9314; 813.81, E818.0
&#9315; 813.91, E825.2

_____ 4. Light-headedness after taking a diazoxide prescription:

&#9312; 780.4, E942.5
&#9313; 386.9, E942.5
&#9314; 780.09
&#9315; 780.4

_____ 5. Select the correct code(s) for a plantar wart due to human papillomavirus infection.

&#9312; 078.19, 079
&#9313; 078.1
&#9314; 079.4
&#9315; 078.12, 079.4

_____ 6. Acute bulbar type I infantile paralysis:

&#9312; 045.0
&#9313; 045.9
&#9314; 045.01
&#9315; 045.91

_____ 7. Which code classifies preinvasive cancer of the female breast, upper-inner quadrant?

① 239.3
② 198.81
③ 217
④ 233.0

_____ 8. Screening test to rule out a suspected malignant neoplasm of the lung:

① V76.0
② V74.1
③ V76.0, 162.9
④ 162.9, V76.0

_____ 9. Select the correct code for chronic viral hepatitis B.

① 070.49
② 070.32
③ 070.3
④ 070

_____ 10. A patient has been diagnosed with Burkitt's tumor in the groin and the neck. Select the correct code(s).

① 200.8
② 200.25, 200.21
③ 200.20
④ 200.28

_____ 11. Select the correct code(s) for glaucoma and brittle type II diabetes.

① 250.00, 365.44
② 250.50
③ 250.50, 365.44
④ 250.40

_____ 12. Which of the following codes is correct for a diagnosis of abnormal coagulation profile?

① 790.92
② 286.9
③ 286.90
④ 776.0

_____ 13. Select the correct code for factor VIII deficiency.

① 286.4
② 286.0
③ 286.2
④ 286.3

_____ 14. Which of the following correctly codes senile dementia with confusion and depression?

① 290.0
② 290.2, 290.3
③ 290.3, 290.21
④ 290.41, 290.43

_____ 15. Select the correct code for recurrent manic-depressive disorder.

① 296.0
② 296.1
③ 296.14
④ 296.10

_____ 16. Choose the codes that correctly describe meningitis due to St. Louis encephalitis.

① 321.2
② 321.2, 062.3
③ 062.3, 321.2
④ 323.4

_____ 17. Lesions of the lateral and medial popliteal nerves:

① 355.2
② 355.3, 355.4
③ 724.3
④ 353.3, 353.4

_____ 18. An elderly female patient has been diagnosed with glaucomatous subcapsular flecks and wide-angle glaucoma. Select the correct code(s).

① 365.10, 366.31
② 365.11
③ 365.10
④ 366.31, 365.10

_____ 19. A 43-year-old male patient receives a diagnosis of essential hypertension and chronic endocarditis. Choose the correct code(s).

① 401.1, 424.90
② 402.9, 424.90
③ 410.0
④ 401.9, 424.90

_____ 20. A 64-year-old female patient is readmitted to the hospital for evaluation of an acute myocardial infarction that occurred 3 weeks ago.

① 410.9
② 410.90
③ 410.91
④ 410.92

_____ 21. Select the correct code(s) for a diagnosis of acute influenzal myocarditis.

&#9312;  487.8, 422.0
&#9313;  422.0, 487.8
&#9314;  422.90, 487.8
&#9315;  487.8, 422.90

_____ 22. The patient's diagnosis is vesicoureteral reflux with nephropathy and chronic pyelonephritis due to *Escherichia coli* infection. Select the correct code(s).

&#9312;  593.70, 590.00, 041.4
&#9313;  590.00, 041.4
&#9314;  593.73, 590.00, 041.4
&#9315;  590.00, 041.4, 593.73

_____ 23. Purulent pleurisy with bronchocutaneous fistula due to a bacterial infection:

&#9312;  511.0, 041.9
&#9313;  510.0, 041.9
&#9314;  510.0
&#9315;  510.0, 510.9, 041.9

_____ 24. Choose the codes that properly classify ulcerative and acute gingivitis.

&#9312;  523.1, 523.0
&#9313;  523.4, 523.1
&#9314;  522.6, 523.0
&#9315;  523.00, 523.10

_____ 25. The patient is diagnosed with a recurrent gangrenous ventral hernia. Select the correct code(s).

&#9312;  551.21
&#9313;  553.21, 785.4
&#9314;  785.4, 553.21
&#9315;  551.21, 785.4

_____ 26. Diverticulosis and diverticulitis of the small intestine with bleeding:

&#9312;  562.01
&#9313;  562.03
&#9314;  562.01, 578.9
&#9315;  562.02, 562.03

_____ 27. A 58-year-old male patient has stenosis of the vesicourethral orifice and urinary incontinence. Select the correct code(s).

&#9312;  596.0, 625.6
&#9313;  596.0, 788.30
&#9314;  596.0
&#9315;  753.6, 788.30

_____ 28. A female infant 25 days old is light for her age, weighed 1200 grams at birth, and has dry peeling skin. Select the correct code(s).

① 764.14, 764.9
② 765.04
③ 764.04
④ 764.14

_____ 29. A pregnant patient in the twentieth week of gestation experiences bleeding.

① 640.9
② 640.90
③ 640.95
④ 640.80

_____ 30. Select the correct code(s) for acute pericardial effusion and chronic uremia.

① 420.0, 585
② 420.0, 586
③ 585.9, 420.0
④ 788.9

_____ 31. A patient's diagnosis is periostitis and acute osteomyelitis of the femur. Choose the correct code(s).

① 730.2
② 730.25
③ 730.36
④ 730.05

_____ 32. An infant is diagnosed with spina bifida and hydrocephalus; its spinal column at C1 and C2 did not close during fetal development. Which code is correct?

① 741.00
② 741.01
③ 741.91
④ 741.03

_____ 33. Eighteen hours following the delivery of her baby, a female patient suffers atonic hemorrhage. Choose the correct code.

① 666.1
② 666.0
③ 666.14
④ 666.10

_____ 34. A 24-year-old female patient has positive result from an HIV test; she is asymptomatic at the present. Which code is correct?

① 042
② V73.89
③ V08
④ V01.7

_____ 35. A patient presents to the emergency room in some distress, complaining of chest pain in the vicinity of the heart. The correct code is:

① 786.5
② 786.50
③ 786.51
④ 786.59

_____ 36. After an accident in which a car tire blows up, a patient suffers injuries to the saphenous vein and popliteal artery and vein. Select the correct codes.

① 904.3, 904.41, 904.42, E921.8
② 904.3, 904.40, E921.8
③ E921.8, 904.3, 904.40
④ 904.3, 904.41, 904.42

_____ 37. A patient experiences a superficial sunburn on the eyelids. Which is the correct code?

① 941.09, E926.2
② 941.12, E926.2
③ 940.1, E926.2
④ 692.71, E926.2

_____ 38. A patient has gastric hemorrhage following the ingestion of lye. Select the correct code(s).

① 983.2, 578.9
② 983.2, 578.9, E980.6
③ 578.9, 983.2
④ 578.9, E980.6

_____ 39. After having acute poliomyelitis as a child, a patient experiences muscle weakness.

① 728.9, 138
② 138, 728.9
③ 138
④ 728.9

_____ 40. From a fire in a school, a patient has first-degree burns of the back of the hand and third-degree burns of the left foot. Which codes are correct?

① E891.8, 945.32, 944.16
② 945.32, 944.16, 948.21, E891.3
③ 945.32, 944.16, 948.21
④ 945.32, 944.16, E891.3

# Part 2 CPT and HCPCS

CPT, a publication of the American Medical Association, contains the codes mandated by HIPAA for professional services and procedures. These CPT codes also make up Level I of the Health Care Common Procedure Coding System (HCPCS) of the Centers for Medicare and Medicaid Services. Level II of HCPCS has codes to identify products, supplies, and services not covered in CPT. HCPCS is the HIPAA-mandated code set for Medicare and Medicaid services, and its Level II codes are also used by private payers.

The CPT manual contains three types of codes. Category I codes, which make up most of the book, describe the procedures and services that are commonly used in medical practice and performed by physicians in the United States. Category II codes are used for performance-measurement tracking. Category III codes are assigned as temporary codes for emerging technology, services, and procedures.

HCPCS and CPT codes are updated annually, except for Category II and III codes, which are updated twice a year. The CPT and HCPCS code sets are released midyear and take effect on January 1 of each year. HIPAA requires the correct codes to be used as of their effective date for reporting to all payers, both government and private.

CPT's main text, which contains the Category I codes, has these six sections of codes:

- Evaluation and Management      Codes 99201–99499
- Anesthesia                     Codes 00100–01999
- Surgery                        Codes 10040–69990
- Radiology                      Codes 70010–79999
- Pathology and Laboratory       Codes 80047–89398
- Medicine                       Codes 90281–99607

CPT codes have five digits (with no decimals) followed by a descriptor, which is a brief explanation of the procedure. Although CPT codes are grouped into sections, such as surgery, codes from any section can be used by all types of physicians. For example, a cardiologist would use codes from the Evaluation and Management Section when assessing a patient's suitability for a vascular procedure.

# Locating Correct Codes

Medical coders follow a series of steps to choose correct procedure codes.

## Step 1.

## Determine the Procedures and Services Performed during the Encounter

The procedures and services performed during the patient's encounter with the provider are documented in the patient's medical record. The main procedure(s) provides the descriptor to be coded first. Additional services or procedures are then coded.

## Step 2.

## Locate the Descriptor in the Index and Verify the Code Selection in the Main Text

### Index

The index is used to find the descriptive term for the main procedure. The main terms in the index are printed in boldface type. The procedure may be listed more than once under these types of main terms:

- The name of the procedure or service
- The name of the organ or other anatomical site
- The name of the condition
- A synonym or an eponym for the term
- The abbreviation for the term.

The index entry provides a pointer to the correct code range in the main text. Using the CPT index makes the process of selecting procedural codes more efficient. If the term is not located under a particular procedure or service, look next under alternate terms, such as *excision* instead of *removal*. Check also under the anatomical name or condition.

### Main Text

The main text listing is reviewed to verify the selection of the correct code. Each of its six sections lists codes and descriptions under subsection headings. These headings group procedures or services, body systems, anatomical sites, or tests and examinations. Following these headings are additional subgroups of procedures, systems, or sites. The section, subsection, and code number ranges contained on a particular page are shown at the top of each page, making it easier to locate a code.

Note that each section begins with guidelines for the use of its codes. The guidelines cover definitions and items unique to the section, as well as special notes about its structure or the rules for its use. The guidelines must be carefully studied and followed for correct coding.

CPT uses a semicolon when a common part of a main entry applies to entries that follow. The descriptor that appears before the semicolon is the first part of a complete procedural description. Each descriptor that follows

## CATEGORY I CODE SECTIONS

| Section | Definition of Codes | Structure | Key Guidelines |
|---------|---------------------|-----------|----------------|
| Evaluation and Management | Physicians' services that are performed to determine the best course for patient care | Organized by place, type, and level of service | • New or established patients; other definitions<br>• Unlisted services, special reports<br>• Selecting an E/M service level |
| Anesthesia | Anesthesia services done by or supervised by a physician; includes general, regional, and supplementation local anesthesia | Organized by body site | • Time-based<br>• Services covered (bundled) in codes<br>• Unlisted services, special reports<br>• Qualifying circumstances codes |
| Surgery | Surgical procedures performed by physicians | Organized by body system and then body site, followed by procedural groups | • Surgical package definition<br>• Follow-up care definition<br>• Add-on codes<br>• Separate procedures<br>• Subsection notes<br>• Unlisted services, special reports |
| Radiology | Radiology services done by or supervised by a physician | Organized by type of procedure followed by body site | • Unlisted services, special reports<br>• Supervision and interpretation (professional vs. technical components) |
| Pathology and Laboratory | Pathology and laboratory services done by physicians or by physician-supervised technicians | Organized by type of procedure | • Complete procedure<br>• Panels<br>• Unlisted services, special reports |
| Medicine | Evaluation, therapeutic, and diagnostic procedures done or supervised by a physician | Organized by type of service or procedure | • Subsection notes<br>• Multiple procedures reported separately<br>• Add-on codes<br>• Separate procedures<br>• Unlisted services, special reports |

the semicolon adds a unique word or words to complete the description. Note that the first letter of the common descriptor is capitalized, but the unique descriptors after the semicolon are not. Usually, the first unique entry appears in the same descriptor as the common part, and the other unique entries are indented below the first.

## Resequenced Codes

As new procedures are widely adopted, CPT has encountered situations where there are not enough numbers left in a particular numerical sequence of codes for all the new items. Also, at times codes need to be regrouped into related procedures for clarity.

To handle this need, the AMA decided to resequence codes rather than renumbering and moving them. *Resequencing* means to display the codes in CPT out of numerical order so that they can be grouped according to the relationships among the code descriptions. It permits out-of-sequence code numbers to be inserted under the previous key procedural terms without having to renumber and move the entire list of related codes.

Codes that are resequenced are listed two times in CPT. First, they are listed in their original numeric position with the note that the code is now out of numerical sequence and refers the user to the code range containing the resequenced code and description.

## Step 3.
## Determine the Need for Modifiers

A CPT modifier is a two-digit number that may be appended to most five-digit procedure codes. Modifiers are used to communicate special circumstances involved with a procedure that are not adequately covered by the code descriptor. A modifier indicates to payers that the procedure was altered in some way that may affect the level of that code's reimbursement.

# Applying Coding Guidelines

The CPT section of the *Medical Coding Workbook for Physician Practices and Facilities* is designed to build your skill in applying CPT coding guidelines. While following the organization of CPT, each section or subsection begins with a *Coding Tip* that explains important procedural coding rules, processes, or information. Some of these tips apply just to the particular CPT section in which you are studying them, and others apply globally when coding procedures and services. After completion of all the exercises in this part, you will know how to apply guidelines concerning:

- Modifier selection
- Bilateral and unilateral codes
- New and established patients
- Level of evaluation and management service—history, examination, and medical decision making
- Consultation versus referral
- Problems treated during preventive medicine services
- Anesthesia modifiers and qualifying circumstances codes
- Codes for add-on procedures
- Package codes and global periods
- Codes that include conscious sedation
- Radiological supervision and interpretation
- Surgical procedures include diagnostic procedures
- Separate procedures
- Procedures performed using various techniques or approaches
- Biopsies
- The obstetric package
- Procedures exempt from the -51 modifier
- Operating microscope
- Unlisted procedures and special reports
- Panels
- Injections
- Cardiac catheterization
- Category II code updates
- Category III code updates
- Locating correct HCPCS codes

NAME _____

# Modifiers

A CPT modifier indicates that a procedure was different from the standard description, but not in a way that changed the definition or required a different code. Modifiers are used mainly when:

- A service or procedure was performed more than once or by more than one physician.
- A service or procedure has been increased or reduced.
- Only part of a procedure was done. For example, some procedures have two parts—a technical component performed by a technician, and a professional component that the physician performed, usually the interpretation and reporting of the results. A modifier is used to show that just one of the parts was done.
- Unusual difficulties occurred during the procedure.

The modifiers are listed in Appendix A of CPT and in Appendix B of this workbook. However, not all CPT modifiers are available for use with every section's codes. Some modifiers apply only to certain sections.

Payers require the hyphen and the two-digit modifier to be appended to the CPT code. Two or more modifiers may be used with one code to give the most accurate description possible.

## CODING TIP

### Bilateral and Unilateral Codes

Some procedures have a pair of codes, one for a unilateral service and another for a bilateral service. Others are bilateral, applying to both anatomical parts or sections. For example, in the audiology section, the tinnitus assessment code 92625 describes a test of both ears. In other cases, codes are unilateral and require a -50 modifier when performed on both parts or sections.

If a procedure with a bilateral code is performed on just one of the two parts, a modifier is also needed. Use the -52 modifier, reduced services, to show that half the work described by the code was done.

## Provide the correct modifier for each of the following descriptions.

1. multiple modifiers _____

2. distinct procedural service _____

3. unrelated Evaluation and Management service by same physician during a postoperative period _____

4. staged procedure _____

5. assistant surgeon _____

6. discontinued procedure _____

7. repeat procedure by same physician _____

8. unusual anesthesia _____

9. mandated services _____

10. surgical team _____

11. surgeon administers a regional Bier block _____

12. patient hemorrhaged heavily during surgery; procedure took twice as long as typically required to perform _____

13. surgeon repairs the flexor tendon of the foot and excises a ganglion on the fourth toe _____

14. during an operation, a thoracic surgeon provides surgical access to the spine while an orthopedist performs a spinal fusion

_____

15. surgeon provides part of a procedure _____

16. patient is returned to the operating room three hours after surgery because of ruptured sutures _____

17. This patient had been in Vermont skiing where he fractured his tibia. The surgery to repair the tibia was performed in Vermont. The patient was so anxious to get back home that he left the day after surgery and returned to his own orthopedist who did all the follow-up care.

_____

_____

18. After mammography findings of a density in both breasts, a patient undergoes puncture aspiration of a cyst in each breast.

_____

_____

19. A radiologist who is not employed by the hospital provides the reporting function for all x-rays taken at the hospital. What modifier is used to reflect her services?

_____

_____

20. During the performance of a left lung lobectomy, a surgeon discontinues the surgery as he realizes the patient is going into shock during the procedure.

_____

_____

# Evaluation and Management
## Codes 99201–99499

The codes in the Evaluation and Management Section (E/M codes) of CPT cover physicians' services that are performed to determine the best course for patient care. Most codes are organized by the place of service. A few, such as consultations, are grouped by type of service. The subsections are as follows:

Office or Other Outpatient Services

Hospital Observation Services

Hospital Inpatient Services

Consultations

Emergency Department Services

Critical Care Services

Nursing Facility Services

Domiciliary, Rest Home, or Custodial Care Services

Domiciliary, Rest Home, or Home Care Plan Oversight Services

Home Services

Prolonged Services

Case Management Services

Care Plan Oversight Services

Preventive Medicine Services

Non-Face-to-Face Physician Services

Special E/M Services

Newborn Care Services

Inpatient Neonatal Intensive Care Services and Pediatric and Neonatal Critical Care Services

Other E/M Services

Many subsections list different code ranges for new and for established patients. A new patient has not received any professional services from the physician (or from another physician of the same specialty in the same group practice) within the past three years. An established patient has received professional services under those conditions.

In some medical practices, physicians assign E/M codes; in others, medical coders perform this task. In either case, code assignment should always be audited using a careful comparison between the codes that are reported and the procedures that are documented in the patient's medical record.

To select the correct E/M code, follow these eight steps.

# Step 1.
# Determine the Category and Subcategory of Service Based on the Location of Service and the Patient's Status

# Step 2.
# Determine the Extent of the History That Is Documented

The extent of the history that the physician obtains is one of four levels:

- Problem-Focused
- Expanded Problem-Focused
- Detailed
- Comprehensive

These components of history may be documented in the patient medical record:

- History of Present Illness (HPI)
- Review of Systems (ROS)
- Past Medical History (PMH)
- Family History (FH)
- Social History (SH)

The extent of history is determined according to the following table:

| Extent of History | History of Present Illness | Review of Systems | Past/Family/ Social History |
|---|---|---|---|
| PROBLEM-FOCUSED | Brief | None | None |
| EXPANDED PROBLEM-FOCUSED | Brief | Problem-Pertinent | None |
| DETAILED | Extended | Extended | Problem-Pertinent |
| COMPREHENSIVE | Extended | Complete | Complete |

# Step 3.
# Determine the Extent of the Examination That Is Documented

The physician may examine a particular body area or organ system, or conduct a multisystem examination. The examination is categorized as one of four levels:

- Problem-Focused—a limited examination of the affected body area or system
- Expanded Problem-Focused—a limited examination of the affected body area or system and other related areas
- Detailed—an extended examination of the affected body area or system and other related areas
- Comprehensive—a general multisystem examination, or a complete examination of a single organ system

Note that there are guidelines about the categories of examinations that are not printed in CPT. Called the "Documentation Guidelines for Evaluation and

Management Services," they have important details used by physicians and medical coders to categorize the extent of examinations. Two sets of guidelines are currently approved for use, the 1995 and the 1997 versions. The set of guidelines used by the medical practice should be specified and available to medical coders, along with other references.

## Step 4.
## Determine the Complexity of Medical Decision Making (MDM) That Is Documented

The complexity of medical decisions involves how many possible diagnoses or treatment options were considered; how much data (such as test results or previous records) were considered to analyze the patient's problem; and how much risk there is for significant complications, advanced illness, or death. The decisions that the physician makes are categorized as one of four types:

- Straightforward
- Low Complexity
- Moderate Complexity
- High Complexity

| Complexity of Medical Decision Making | Diagnosis Options | Data Reviewed | Risks |
|---|---|---|---|
| STRAIGHTFORWARD | Few | Little or none | Minimal |
| LOW COMPLEXITY | Limited | Limited | Low |
| MODERATE COMPLEXITY | Many | Moderate | Moderate |
| HIGH COMPLEXITY | Extensive | Extensive | High |

## Step 5.
## Analyze the Requirements to Report the Service Level

The descriptor for each E/M code explains the standards for its use. For office visits and most other services to new patients, and for initial care visits, all three of the key component requirements—history, exam, and MDM—generally must be met. For most services for established patients, and for subsequent care visits, two out of three of the key component requirements generally must be met.

## Step 6.
## Review the Nature of the Presenting Problem and the Time Spent with the Patient

Many descriptors mention two additional components: (1) how severe the patient's condition is—referred to as the "nature of the presenting problem"—and (2) how much time the physician typically spends directly treating the patient. These factors, while not the key components, are helpful in selecting the correct service level.

## Step 7.
## Verify That the Documentation Is Complete

Meeting the requirements means that the documentation must contain the record of the physician's work. When an E/M code is assigned, the patient's medical record must contain the clinical details to support it. The history, examination, and medical decision making must be sufficiently documented so that the medical necessity and appropriateness of the service can be understood.

## Step 8.
## Assign the Code

The code that has been selected is assigned. The need for any modifiers, based on the documentation of special circumstances, is also reviewed.

---

### CODING TIP

#### Reimbursement for Consultations Depends on the Payer

A consultation occurs when a second physician provides services requested by the patient's primary physician and then returns the patient to that primary physician, with a written report of findings, to continue care. Referrals, on the other hand, involve the assumption of care by the physician to whom the patient is referred.

Because of suspected misuse of consultation codes, which reimburse at a higher rate than regular visits, CMS has decided not to pay them. Coders coding for Medicare-paid (Original Medicare Plan) visits should use new/established patient codes for office/outpatient consultations and initial/subsequent hospital care codes for inpatient consultations.

---

### CODING TIP

#### Problems Treated during Preventive Medicine Service

An illness or clinical sign of a condition may be found during a routine physical examination that requires the physician to conduct an additional evaluation of the problem. In this case, the preventive medicine service code is reported first, followed by the appropriate E/M code for the new problem, adding the -25 modifier, Significant, Separate E/M Service.

---

# Evaluation and Management
## *continued*

**Provide procedure codes from the Evaluation and Management Section for the following procedures.**

1. initial office visit, 25-year-old male, with boil on back; physician took a brief history, performed a limited examination of the back, and there was little risk of complications and minimal treatment options.

   _____

2. office visit, established patient is a 67-year-old female, with controlled diabetes mellitus, complaining of lack of sensation in her feet; expanded problem-focused history and examination

   _____

3. first hospital visit, admitting physician, comprehensive history, examination, and moderate decision making _____

4. initial office consultation, non-Medicare; detailed history and examination, low complexity medical decision making _____

5. annual comprehensive physical examination for 11-year-old new patient _____

6. medical disability examination by physician employed by state _____

7. hospital visit to previously admitted patient; problem-focused history and examination, 10 minutes spent at bedside _____

8. emergency department service for patient following a car accident; comprehensive history and examination, highly complex decision making _____

9. discharge of patient from nursing home, 45-minute encounter _____

10. home visit for established patient, straightforward case, problem-focused examination _____

11. While hospitalized for surgery, a non-Medicare patient takes a minor fall and hurts his elbow. An orthopedist is called in to consult on the patient to be sure it is a minimal injury. He determines it is a minor problem, and his visit is brief. _____

12. A patient is badly injured in a car accident and is put in an ambulance to get to the emergency department. On the way, his blood pressure drops and he has difficulty breathing. The EMT calls the ED physician who directs the care of the patient until they reach the hospital.

_____

13. A patient is admitted to the hospital in respiratory failure and kidney failure. He is sent to the intensive care unit where the ICU physician works on him for one hour to restore his breathing function and to dialyze him until he is stable.

_____

14. A child who is 25 days old was admitted 2 days ago to the neonatal intensive care unit due to cardiac and respiratory insufficiency. Today his physician is again monitoring his cardiac and respiratory support and reevaluating his status. The child has been under constant supervision by the health care team that is supervised by his physician.

_____

15. An 85-year-old woman fell and broke her hip. The hip has been repaired, but she now needs long-term nursing care. She was admitted to a nursing facility 3 days ago and is being seen today in follow-up. She is regaining movement and has an excellent prognosis.

_____

## In addition to E/M codes, provide modifiers and additional procedure codes if appropriate for the following.

16. comprehensive annual examination for established 65-year-old patient

_____

17. Primary care physician sends a Medicare patient to a cardiologist for an evaluation of a complicated vascular problem; during the hour-long encounter, the specialist performs a comprehensive history and examination of this new patient, and follows up the visit with a written report to the PCP; MDM was moderate.

_____

18. Thoracic surgeon provides a second opinion on the appropriateness of a single bypass procedure as requested by a third-party payer; a detailed history and examination are obtained; MDM is of low complexity.

_____

19. During an annual physical examination, a 45-year-old established patient complains of general tiredness and severe shortness of breath during mild activity; physician performs a detailed cardiovascular assessment with additional detailed history; following complex MDM, the physician also schedules an immediate complete heart study.

_____

# Anesthesia Section

## Codes 00100–01999

The codes in this section of CPT are used to report anesthesia services performed by or supervised by a physician. These services include general and regional anesthesia, as well as supplementation of local anesthesia. A single code covers preoperative evaluation and planning, care during the procedure, and routine postoperative care. The subsections are organized by body site.

---

### CODING TIP

#### Anesthesia Modifiers and Qualifying Circumstances Codes

Because the patient's health affects the difficulty of anesthesia services, a physical status modifier is added to the CPT anesthesia code. The patient's physical status—from P1 to P6—is selected from the listing in the Anesthesia Section Guidelines.

Standard modifiers -22, -23, -32, -51, -53, and -59 are also commonly used with anesthesia codes. Note that modifier -47, Anesthesia by Surgeon, is used by surgeons and appended to a surgical procedure code, not for services performed by anesthesiologists or anesthetists or supervised by surgeons.

Another set of codes, also listed in the guidelines, is used in addition to the procedural codes to report qualifying circumstances such as extreme age or emergency conditions.

---

**Provide the CPT code for each of the following anesthesia services. Do not code a physical status modifier for these services; focus on the anesthesia codes.**
***Hint:*** **All codes are in the Anesthesia Section.**

1. cesarean delivery _____

2. arthroscopic procedures of the hip joint _____

3. transurethral resection of prostate _____

4. breast reconstruction _____

5. heart transplant _____

6. needle biopsy of thyroid _____

7. repair of cleft palate _____

8. cervical spine procedure _____

9. esophageal procedure _____

10. thoracoplasty _____

11. Patient presents with severe vaginal bleeding. Multiple malignant tumors are found, and the patient is scheduled for a radical hysterectomy. Code for the anesthesia. _____

12. A patient is experiencing lower abdominal pain, and her gynecologist suspects there is a problem in her uterus and/or fallopian tubes. He schedules a hysterosalpingography. Code for the injection procedure required to perform the hysterosalpingography. _____

13. Two months ago, this patient had abdominal surgery and now presents with pain in the left lower extremity. Examination reveals an embolus in the femoral artery, and surgery is performed to remove the embolus.

    _____

14. After 6 months of shoulder pain, the patient sees her physician. He examines the patient and is concerned that there may be a tear in the shoulder joint ligament, but he cannot be sure without going in with a scope to examine the area. The diagnostic arthroscopy is performed. Code for the anesthesia. _____

15. A pregnant patient comes in to the hospital in labor. This is her first child, so the obstetrician is aware that her labor may be prolonged. She contacts anesthesia to provide a continuous epidural to cover this patient through her labor and vaginal delivery. _____

## Provide the anesthesia code and a modifier for the following services.

16. procedure on popliteal bursa, patient with mild systemic disease

    _____

17. open procedure, sacroiliac joint, normal patient _____

18. major abdominal vessel procedure for patient with life-threatening

    disease _____

19. plastic repair, cleft lip, six-month-old _____

20. amniocentesis, healthy mother _____

21. spinal fluid shunting procedure on moribund patient _____

22. anesthesia is induced but blepharoplasty is canceled _____

23. amputation, ankle and foot, severely diabetic patient _____

24. emergency room appendectomy _____

25. arthroscopic procedure of knee joint, mildly arthritic patient _____

26. cardiac catheterization for patient with malignant hypertension

    _____

27. removal of donated organs from brain-dead patient _____

28. pneumocentesis, elderly patient _____

# Surgery Section

The Surgery Section of CPT has these subsections:

Integumentary System

Musculoskeletal System

Respiratory System

Cardiovascular System

Hemic and Lymphatic Systems

Mediastinum and Diaphragm

Digestive System

Urinary System

Male Genital System

Intersex Surgery

Female Genital System

Maternity Care and Delivery

Endocrine System

Nervous System

Eye and Ocular Adnexa

Operating Microscope

The Surgery Section Guidelines contain both general information and a listing of the subsections that have unique special instructions. These notes should be carefully read before selecting codes from the procedures that follow them.

Many of the major system subsections are organized anatomically, covering body parts from head to toe. Within this organization, codes are listed in groups of related types of procedures. Typical groupings are:

- Incisions: procedures that involve cutting into, such as those with the ending *-otomy* or *-tomy* (for example, tracheotomy)
- Excisions: procedures that involve surgical removal, such as those with the ending *-ectomy* (for example, lumpectomy). Other terms are biopsy, resection, or removal; radical resection means total excision.
- Introduction or removal, amputation
- Repair/revision/reconstruction (*-orrhaphy, -oplasty*)
- Manipulation or reduction
- Fixation or fusion (*-opexy*)
- Endoscopic or laparoscopic procedures

Many surgical procedures can be performed in more than one way or via more than one approach. Open surgical procedures are performed by creating a surgical incision to access the site. For some of these, the alternative use of the endoscope permits a less invasive procedure. Endoscopic procedures frequently listed in the Surgery Section include laparoscopy, colonoscopy, bronchoscopy, esophagoscopy, and arthroscopy. These procedures are performed using endoscopic equipment. For example, a laparoscope is an endoscope designed to examine the contents of the peritoneum through a small incision. An arthroscope is an endoscope designed to view the interior of a joint. These are diagnostic endoscopic procedures; the instruments are also used for surgical procedures. Other open procedures may be endoscopically assisted. Coders study the terminology used to identify the technique that has been used.

Surgical destruction is usually a part of the surgical procedure and is not listed under a separate grouping.

Two codes for fine needle aspiration are listed before the first surgical subsection. These codes are general and apply to any body system.

# Integumentary System

## Codes 10040–19499

The codes in this subsection of CPT's Surgery Section cover procedures performed on the integumentary system, including the skin, subcutaneous and accessory structures, nails, and breast. Integumentary system services also include wound and burn repairs as well as skin grafts.

The guidelines for many groupings of procedures, such as paring, excision, or destruction, indicate which specific services are included. For example, shaving of lesions includes local anesthesia and chemical or electrocauterization of the wound. Such services cannot be reported in addition to the code for the procedure.

---

### CODING TIP

#### Codes for Add-On Procedures

A plus sign (+) next to any code in CPT designates an add-on procedure that is commonly carried out in addition to a primary procedure. Add-on code descriptors usually use phrases such as "each additional" or "list separately in addition to the primary procedure." The add-on codes are also listed in CPT's Appendix D.

In reporting add-on codes, do not list them alone or modify them with a -51 modifier. There are many add-on codes in the Integumentary System subsection; exercises 31–35 provide practice.

---

### Provide the integumentary system codes for the following procedures.

1. simple incision and removal of foreign body, subcutaneous tissue

   _____

2. complicated I&D, abscess _____

3. excision of benign lesion, 0.5-cm diameter, upper arm _____

4. excision of a 2.1-cm benign lesion from the foot _____

5. abrasion of a single lesion _____

6. cervicoplasty _____

7. rhytidectomy of glabellar frown lines _____

8. escharotomy _____

9. breast reduction _____

10. breast reconstruction with free flap _____

11. Patient is having surgery for aberrant breast tissue. Once started, the surgeon determines that a lumpectomy is required, and performs that procedure. _____

12. Patient presents with a 4.1-cm malignant lesion on the nose. Due to the location of the lesion and the depth of the lesion, the surgeon removes it by chemical destruction, instead of excision. _____

13. Patient is being treated for psoriasis. She now has severe psoriasis lesions that have not responded to oral medication. Today her physician will provide steroid injections into nine of those lesions. _____

14. After excision of a malignant lesion, the patient was left with a defect too large to repair by simple closure. The surgeon elected to use a neurovascular pedicle flap to ensure that the defect would have adequate blood supply to heal correctly. _____

15. After observing that a spot on her upper leg had grown bigger, a patient saw her dermatologist. The dermatologist determined that she had a malignant 3.3-cm lesion which he biopsied and excised, followed by a simple closure. _____

## Some of the following procedures require two codes and/or the use of a modifier.

16. excision of malignant lesions, 1.1 cm, upper arm; 0.1 cm, foot _____

17. split graft, 80 sq cm, lower leg, staged procedure on infant _____

18. surgical removal of excess skin and tissue, upper arm and hand _____

19. needle core biopsy of both breasts (not using imaging guidance) ____

20. preparation and insertion of custom breast implant five days after mastectomy _____

## Hint: Each of the following procedures requires add-on codes.

21. abrasion, nine lesions _____

22. application of 200 sq cm skin xenograft _____

23. laser destruction of four premalignant lesions _____

24. debridement of infected skin, 18 percent of body surface _____

25. complex repair of wound on trunk, 12 cm _____

# Musculoskeletal System

## Codes 20000–29999

The codes in this subsection of CPT's Surgery Section cover procedures performed on the musculoskeletal system. General procedures, such as wound treatments, excision services, and grafts, are listed first. Codes are then grouped by body site, beginning with the head and ending with the foot. Each body site has the same organization: incision, excision, introduction/removal, repair/revision/reconstruction, fracture/dislocation, manipulation, arthrodesis (fusion or fixation), amputation, and other procedures. Casts/strapping and endoscopy/arthroscopy are the final code groups in the subsection.

---

### CODING TIP

#### Package Codes and Global Periods

A package is a group of related procedures and/or services included under a single code. As defined in CPT, a surgical package includes the operation itself, local anesthesia (injection of a metacarpal/digital block or topical anesthesia), and all routine follow-up services. For example, in the musculoskeletal subsection, surgical package codes include the application and the removal of the first cast or traction device. Payers often add some preoperative services to their definition of a package.

Payers set a global period—a certain length of time for which the expected services are to be provided—for each package. During a global period, no packaged service is reimbursed in addition to the fee for the package code. After the global period ends, all services that are provided can be reported.

Some types of services are not considered to be routine follow-up and are reported during the global period. For example, complications or recurrences that arise after therapeutic surgical procedures are reported with appropriate modifiers (such as for repeat or related surgical procedures). Care for other illnesses, injuries, or conditions that are unrelated to the surgical procedure are also separately reported. In these cases, use a -24 or -79 modifier when an E/M service or a procedure performed during the global period is not related to the package and should be paid. Following a diagnostic procedure, services not related to the recovery from that procedure may be reported, even though the care may be related to the patient's underlying condition.

---

## Provide the musculoskeletal system codes for the following procedures.

1. removal of body cast applied by another physician _____

2. primary repair of ruptured Achilles tendon _____

3. tendon sheath incision _____

4. closed treatment of fractured ulnar shaft _____

5. complete wrist arthrodesis _____

6. humeral osteotomy _____

7. closed treatment of sesamoid fracture _____

8. open treatment of talus fracture _____

9. I&D of foot bursa _____

10. elbow joint arthrodesis _____

11. lateral elbow tenotomy, open with bone debridement _____

12. distal humeral sequestrectomy _____

13. reinsertion of spinal fixation device _____

14. posterior arthrodesis for spinal deformity with cast _____

15. radial and ulnar osteotomy _____

16. amputation of tip of right thumb with direct closure _____

17. percutaneous skeletal fixation of posterior pelvic ring dislocation

    _____

18. trocar biopsy of rib _____

19. anterior capsulorrhaphy, transfer of coracoid process _____

20. surgical removal of prepatellar bursa _____

21. Nine months after a humeral fracture repair, a patient returns to his physician with pain in the fracture area. Unfortunately the patient had not returned prior to this time for fracture care follow-up and now has a nonunion of the humeral fracture. The surgeon does an iliac graft to repair the nonunion. _____

22. Patient with osteoarthritis has been treated medically for the erosion of cartilage in the hip for over 5 years. After extensive discussion with the surgeon, the patient agrees to have a total hip replacement procedure performed. The surgeon explains that the surgery requires replacement of the acetabulum and the proximal femur with a prosthesis. _____

23. After a bicycle fall, a patient sought treatment for right hip pain. The orthopedist determined that the acetabulum (hip socket) was fractured, but that it could be treated with manipulation and skeletal traction, rather than doing an open procedure to correct the fracture. _____

# Musculoskeletal System *continued*

24. Concerned about the spread of the patient's osteomyelitis of the proximal humerus, the orthopedic surgeon performed a craterization of that bone in hopes of stopping any further spread of the infection.

    _____

25. A patient whose back was strapped due to severe muscle spasms fell off a ladder and was in extreme pain. It was late in the evening, and the patient went to the emergency department for evaluation and treatment. After removing the strapping that was already in place, the ED physician was able to determine that the patient had wrenched his back again, but there was no dislocation or fracture. The ED physician put replacement strapping on the patient and indicated that the patient should see his orthopedist in the morning for follow-up care.

    _____

## Some of the following procedures require two codes and/or the use of a modifier.

26. Keller procedure, left and right halluces _____

27. surgical exploration of chest wound with debridement and removal of foreign body _____

28. arthrodesis of sacroiliac joint, graft harvested _____

29. talectomy provided during global period of previous unrelated surgery

    _____

30. medial and lateral meniscectomy _____

31. closed treatment of ankle dislocation under anesthesia with percutaneous skeletal fixation _____

32. epiphyseal arrest of distal femur, proximal tibia, and proximal fibula

    _____

33. closed treatment of dislocated sternoclavicular joint and patella

    _____

34. synovial biopsy and diagnostic arthroscopy of hip _____

35. surgical arthroscopy, ankle, with removal of foreign body _____

# Respiratory System
## Codes 30000–32999

The codes in this surgical subsection of CPT cover procedures performed on the respiratory system. Codes are grouped by body site: the nose, accessory sinuses, larynx, trachea and bronchi, and lungs and pleura. Each body site is organized by the type of procedure as appropriate: incision, excision, repair, introduction, and endoscopic. Each site's procedural guidelines specify the included services.

---

### CODING TIP

#### Codes That Include Conscious Sedation

In CPT, the symbol ⊙ (a bullet inside a circle) next to a code means that conscious sedation is a part of the procedure performed by the operating physician and should not be additionally coded. Conscious sedation is a moderate, drug-induced depression of consciousness during which patients can respond to verbal commands. This type of sedation is typically used with procedures such as bronchoscopies.

---

**Provide the respiratory system codes for the following procedures. Include any necessary modifiers.**

1. maxillectomy _____

2. maxillary sinus irrigation _____

3. total laryngectomy _____

4. laryngoplasty, cricoid split _____

5. simple revision of tracheostoma _____

6. cervical tracheoplasty _____

7. parietal pleurectomy _____

8. extrapleural thoracoplasty _____

9. complex surgical removal of dermoid cyst from nose _____

10. lateral rhinotomy to remove object from nose _____

Some of the following procedures require two codes. *Hint:* For endoscopic procedures, read the notes before this code group carefully.

11. surgical thoracoscopy with excisions of pericardial and mediastinal

    cysts _____

12. surgical nasal/sinus endoscopy with maxillary antrostomy _____

13. planned tracheostomy on infant _____

14. hematoma drainage from nasal septum _____

15. laser destruction of two intranasal lesions, internal approach _____

16. sinusotomy, three paranasal sinuses _____

17. bilateral nasal evaluation using endoscope _____

18. direct diagnostic laryngoscopy and tracheoscopy with operating micro-

    scope _____

19. diagnostic nasal/sinus endoscopy with sphenoid sinusoscopy and
    inspection of interior nasal cavity, sphenoethmoid recess and turbinates

    _____

20. turbinate excision followed by intranasal antrotomy _____

21. A neonate, born several hours ago, develops respiratory distress and
    requires emergency endotracheal intubation. _____

22. A patient comes to the emergency department after a motor vehicle
    accident. The patient did not wear a seat belt and was injured when
    he hit the steering wheel. The doctors determined that his lung was
    deflated as a result of air accumulated in the thoracic cavity. They did a
    thoracentesis and inserted a tube to allow for the air to escape and the
    lung to reinflate. _____

23. After determining that the patient had developed lung cancer in both
    lobes of the right lung, the thoracic surgeon removed two lobes due to
    the extent of the cancerous tissue. _____

24. Years of chronic sinusitis had created a severe blockage of the ethmoid
    sinus cavity on the left side, discovered on CT exam. A sinus endos-
    copy was performed to remove tissue from the ethmoid sinus both
    anterior and posterior. _____

25. A patient with asthma since childhood now presents with increased dif-
    ficulty breathing. A CT scan indicates an abnormality in the right mid-
    dle lobe. To finalize this patient's diagnosis, a diagnostic bronchoscopy
    is performed. _____

# Cardiovascular System

## Codes 33010–37799

The codes in this surgical subsection of CPT cover procedures performed on the cardiovascular system. Codes are grouped in two large sections, the heart and pericardium followed by the arteries and veins. Cardiac procedures include placement of pacemakers/pacing cardioverter-defibrillators, surgery on the heart valves, and coronary artery bypass.

Many cardiac procedures include related procedures. For example, coronary artery bypasses include taking arteries or the saphenous vein graft from other body sites. Arterial and venous procedures, such as aneurysm repair, angioplasty, and catheter placement, include establishing blood inflow and outflow as well as arteriograms that the surgeon performs.

---

### CODING TIP

*Radiological Supervision and Interpretation*

Often the physician supervises and interprets radiological imaging such as x-rays in the course of performing surgery. When the physician provides radiological supervision and interpretation (S&I), a professional component modifier (-26) is attached to the radiology code that is reported with the surgery codes.

The appropriate radiology code or code range is mentioned with the associated surgery codes in CPT. If more than one code is mentioned, the coder turns to the Radiology Section and examines the listed codes to select the correct option. In some cases, separate codes are listed for the professional and the technical components of the service.

Note that the professional component modifier is not used if the physician owns the equipment, provides the supplies, and employs the technicians used for the radiological imaging. In that case, the physician is providing the complete service, and the modifier is not appropriate.

---

**Provide the cardiovascular system codes for the following procedures. Include any necessary modifiers.**

1. removal of permanent pacemaker pulse generator _____

2. mitral valve valvotomy, closed heart _____

3. coronary artery bypass using single venous graft _____

4. myocardial resection _____

5. repair of complete atrioventricular canal _____

6. saphenopopliteal vein anastomosis _____

7. carotid thromboendarterectomy _____

8. exploration of femoral artery _____

9. intravenous introduction of intracatheter _____

10. closure of ventricular septal defect _____

11. insertion of implantable intraarterial infusion pump _____

12. pericardiectomy with cardiopulmonary bypass _____

13. insertion of transvenous electrode for dual chamber pacing cardioverter-

    defibrillator; initial insertion done 20 days earlier _____

14. aortic suture repair _____

15. repair of transposed great arteries by aortic pulmonary artery

    reconstruction _____

16. pulmonary artery embolectomy _____

17. sinus of Valsalva aneurysm repair with cardiopulmonary bypass

    _____

18. ligation of secondary varicose veins, left and right legs _____

19. repair by division of patent ductus ateriosus in 10-year-old

    _____

20. ring insertion and valvuloplasty, tricuspid valve _____

### The following procedures may require two codes and/or the use of modifiers.

21. subcutaneous removal of pacing cardioverter-defibrillator pulse genera-

    tor, electrodes removed by thoracotomy _____

22. subsequent pericardiocentesis with radiological S&I _____

23. revision of skin pocket for pacing cardioverter-defibrillator

    _____

24. aortic valve replacement using a homograft valve with cardiopulmonary

    bypass _____

25. coronary artery bypass with one arterial graft and three venous grafts

    _____

# Cardiovascular System *continued*

26. carotid and axillary-axillary arterial bypass with venous grafts

   _____

27. radiological S&I for percutaneous transluminal balloon angioplasty

   _____

28. excision of infected abdominal graft, surgical care only _____

29. central venous catheter placed percutaneously in adult _____

30. routine venipuncture _____

## Code the following case studies.

31. Patient with two blocked coronary arteries is scheduled for coronary artery bypass grafting; however, due to sudden tachycardia a single chamber temporary pacemaker is inserted to stabilize the patient, and the bypass surgery is rescheduled for the next day. Code for the temporary pacemaker insertion.

   _____

32. Patient presents for replacement of his pulmonary valve which was determined to have a congenital anomaly. During the surgery the patient develops ventricular tachycardia, and the operation is discontinued.

   _____

33. Patient is examined due to shortness of breath, and angiography reveals an embolus in the pulmonary artery. A surgeon is called in to perform an embolectomy of the pulmonary artery. Code for the surgery.

   _____

34. Patient is placed on heart/lung bypass, and the main pulmonary artery is opened in order to remove the blockage and interior lining of the artery. The artery is then sutured closed, and the pulmonary endarterectomy is accomplished.

   _____

35. Patient with a descending thoracic aneurysm is scheduled for surgery. Despite the new endovascular procedures available to treat aortic aneurysms, this patient's aneurysm is not amenable to the endovascular treatment and will have to undergo an open repair of the descending aorta using a Dacron graft.

   _____

NAME _____

# Hemic and Lymphatic Systems; Mediastinum and Diaphragm

## Codes 38100–39599

Codes in these two surgical subsections of CPT cover procedures involving the spleen, bone marrow or stem cell transplantation, lymph nodes and lymphatic channels, the mediastinum, and the diaphragm.

---

### CODING TIP

#### Surgical Procedures Include Diagnostic Procedures

As a general guideline, surgical procedures include diagnostic procedures. When a diagnostic procedure is the only service, it is reported. When the diagnostic procedure is followed by a surgical procedure, the diagnostic service is not reported. For example, a procedure such as a peritoneoscopy (laparoscopy examination of the peritoneum) to view and diagnose a condition is reported. However, if the diagnostic examination is followed by surgical laparoscopy (through the same scope and during the same surgical session), the diagnostic procedure cannot be separately reported. Note that a diagnostic laparoscopy as a separate procedure is located in the Digestive System subsection, code 49320.

---

**Provide codes for the following procedures. Include any necessary modifiers. In some cases, more than one code is required.**

1.  extensive drainage of lymphadenitis _____

2.  injection procedure for identification of sentinel node _____

3.  laceration repair, diaphragm _____

4.  mediastinoscopy _____

5.  needle biopsy of lymph node _____

6.  axillary excision of cystic hygroma _____

7.  pelvic lymphadenectomy _____

8.  laparoscopic splenectomy _____

9.  total splenectomy _____

10. autologous stem cell transplantation _____

11. injection for lymphangiography _____

12. repair of chronic traumatic diaphragmatic hernia _____

13. lymphangiotomy _____

14. insertion of cannula in thoracic duct _____

15. mediastinotomy with removal of object via cervical approach

   _____

16. injection procedure for splenoportography with radiological S&I

   _____

17. injection procedure for bilateral pelvic/abdominal lymphangiography

   with radiological S&I _____

18. An oncologist recommends that the patient undergo a procedure to
   determine what stage the cancer is in. The surgeon performs a limited
   lymphadenectomy of the aortic and splenic lymph nodes for staging.

   _____

   _____

19. Patient was in a car accident and suffered intraabdominal blunt trauma.
   Upon examination, the physician determined that the spleen had been
   lacerated or ruptured, and surgery was scheduled. A repair of the ruptured spleen was performed. The surgeon also did a partial splenectomy due to other damage found.

   _____

   _____

20. A 50-year-old patient who had a mastectomy 3 years ago now comes in
   with lumps under her arms and on her chest. Both a complete axillary
   lymphadenectomy and a regional thoracic lymphadenectomy must be
   performed.

   _____

   _____

# Digestive System
## Codes 40490–49999

The codes in this surgical subsection of CPT cover procedures performed on the digestive system. Codes are grouped by body site: lips, mouth, pharynx, esophagus, stomach, intestines, rectum, anus, liver, biliary tract, pancreas, and abdomen. Each body site is organized by the type of procedure, such as excision and repair.

Endoscopic procedures are listed under the esophagus, intestines, rectum, anus, and biliary tract. In keeping with coding principles, a surgical endoscopic procedure includes a diagnostic endoscopic procedure.

---

### CODING TIP

#### *Separate Procedures*

Some surgical code descriptors in CPT are followed by the words *separate procedure* in parentheses. These procedures are usually integral parts of the major procedure performed during an operation and therefore are not reported.

In some situations, however, a separate procedure is not done with the major procedure. It is performed alone and coded in the normal way. When a separate procedure is done along with other procedures but for a separate purpose, it may be reported in addition to the major operation code. In this case, the -59 modifier is attached to the separate procedure code to show that it is not a part of another procedure and is distinct and independent.

---

### Provide codes for the following procedures. Include any necessary modifiers. In some cases, more than one code is required.

1. resection of 50 percent of lip _____

2. repair of sliding inguinal hernia _____

3. insertion of peritoneal-venous shunt _____

4. exploratory laparotomy _____

5. removal of pancreatic calculus _____

6. cholecystectomy _____

7. portoenterostomy _____

8. wedge biopsy of liver _____

9. excision of Meckel's diverticulum _____

10. gastroduodenostomy _____

11. frenotomy _____

12. palate resection, repeated procedure by same physician _____

13. secondary adenoidectomy, 10-year-old patient _____

14. near total esophagectomy w/pharyngogastrostomy (w/o thoracotomy)

15. percutaneous placement of gastrostomy tube w/radiological S&I

    _____

16. endoscopic placement of gastrostomy tube w/radiological S&I _____

17. simple ileostomy revision done during same operative session as pha-

    rangeal wound suture _____

18. partial colectomy with ileostomy and creation of mucofistula _____

19. excision of ruptured appendix _____

20. diagnostic and surgical flexible colonoscopy past the splenic flexure

    and tumor removal by bipolar cautery _____

21. The physician does an endoscopic diagnostic evaluation of the patient's
    esophagus and stomach. The scope does not go beyond the cardia of
    the stomach.

    _____

22. Due to a patient's encroaching tumor, the surgeon removes half of the
    patient's tongue (hemiglossectomy).

    _____

23. Patient comes in 1 year after repair of his right and left incarcerated fem-
    oral hernias with a recurrence of that condition. The surgeon schedules
    surgery to repair this recurrent problem. Code for the surgery.

    _____

24. The patient's esophageal cancer has made it almost impossible for him
    to eat normally, and he is becoming malnourished. His physician rec-
    ommends laparoscopically creating an opening into the jejunum (2nd
    portion of the small intestine) to allow for placement of a feeding tube.
    A laparoscopic jejunostomy is performed.

    _____

25. As a result of spasms in the esophagus, the patient is unable to swallow.
    The physician will need a greater than 35-mm balloon dilator to allevi-
    ate this patient's difficulty. Radiologic supervision and interpretation are
    provided via fluoroscopy using the hospital's equipment.

    _____

# Urinary System

## Codes 50010–53899

The codes in this surgical subsection of CPT cover procedures performed on the urinary system. Codes for the kidneys, ureters, bladder, and urethra are listed by the type of procedure. Different codes for males and females are indicated in some bladder and urethra procedures.

Many procedures involving the urinary system involve the use of a laparoscope or an endoscope. They include renal and ureteral laparoscopy and endoscopic procedures, cystoscopy (to view or treat the bladder), urethroscopy (to view or treat the urethra), and cystourethroscopy (using both the cystoscope and the urethroscope to view or treat the urinary collecting system). Therapeutic (surgical) procedures include diagnostic procedures as well as other listed procedures.

---

### CODING TIP

#### Procedures Performed Using Various Techniques or Approaches

In researching codes in CPT, it is useful to be aware that some procedures are performed using different techniques. For example, a sling operation for stress incontinence may be performed as a surgical repair or laparoscopically. Some procedures are done by more than one method. For example, injections can be subcutaneous/intramuscular, intraarterial, or intravenous, each having a code. Carefully examine the description of the procedure to determine which technique or approach has been used before researching the code.

---

**Provide codes for the following procedures. Include any necessary modifiers. In some cases, more than one code is required.**

1. ureterotomy _____

2. ureteroplasty _____

3. ureteral endoscopy through established ureterostomy _____

4. first-stage urethroplasty _____

5. drainage, deep periurethral abscess _____

6. cystourethroscopy with double-J type stent _____

7. closure of cystostomy _____

8. EMG studies of urethral sphincter _____

9. trocar bladder aspiration _____

10. simple bladder irrigation _____

11. ureteroileal conduit and Bricker operation _____

12. laparoscopic nephrectomy _____

13. percutaneous needle renal biopsy with radiological S&I (fluoroscopy)

    _____

14. complicated Foley Y-pyeloplasty _____

15. renal endoscopy through nephrotomy _____

16. completion (second stage) of transurethral prostate resection *Hint:*
    Include a modifier. _____

17. cystourethroscopy with fulguration of 3.0-cm bladder tumor _____

18. unilateral ureteroneocystostomy and cystourethroplasty _____

19. transurethral resection, obstructive tissue, 18 months after a TURP

    _____

20. discontinued contact laser vaporization of prostate _____

21. A urologist pulverizes a patient's kidney stones in the right kidney via
    lithotripsy (using shock waves directed through a water cushion). Over
    the next several days/weeks, the fragments will pass harmlessly through
    the urinary system. _____

22. A patient has been diagnosed with kidney failure and will need to go
    on dialysis until a kidney transplant is possible. Due to various difficul-
    ties with the patient's existing kidneys, both must be removed prior to
    the transplant. Code for their removal. _____

23. A urologist needs to examine both ureters and the bladder. She inserts
    a scope into the ureter(s) making an incision in the opening of the ure-
    ters to the bladder (meatotomy) and completes the examination.

    _____

24. A 70-year-old patient was seen for chronic urinary urgency. The urolo-
    gist's examination revealed an enlarged prostate that was most likely
    the cause of the problem. Testing determined that the patient did not
    have prostate cancer, and drug therapy was prescribed initially. The
    patient's problem was not alleviated, and surgery was recommended.
    The urologist performed an electrosurgical resection of the prostate,
    using a transurethral approach and internal urethrotomy._____

25. After having given birth to four children and having a hysterectomy
    performed in her fifties, the 65-year-old patient presents today because
    she has problems retaining her urine when walking, sneezing, or
    coughing. She is embarrassed and wants the problem corrected. Her
    urologist recommends a sling operation to give her bladder support,
    and he recommends doing it laparoscopically. The patient agrees. Code
    for the surgery that will be performed. _____

# Male Genital System; Intersex Surgery

## Codes 54000–55980

The codes in the male genital system surgical subsection of CPT cover procedures performed on the male genital system. Codes for the penis, testis, epididymis, tunica vaginalis, scrotum, vas deferens, spermatic cord, seminal vesicles, and prostate are listed by type of procedure. Intersex codes cover male-to-female and female-to-male operative procedures.

---

### CODING TIP

*Biopsies*

Codes for biopsies are located in many of the surgical subsections. Biopsies are performed with a number of different techniques, such as needle core, punch, incisional, or fine needle aspiration. In general, biopsies of all types follow the coding principle that surgical procedures include diagnostic procedures. If a biopsy is the only service performed, it is reported. As a general rule, however, if more extensive surgery is performed in addition to the biopsy, then the biopsy procedure is not reported with the major surgical procedure. Biopsies are often separate procedures in CPT.

---

**Provide codes for the following procedures. Include any necessary modifiers. In some cases, more than one code is required.**

1. testicular injury repair _____

2. bilateral simple orchiectomy _____

3. bilateral vasectomy _____

4. complicated vesiculotomy _____

5. laparoscopic orchiopexy _____

6. radical perineal prostatectomy _____

7. excision of Mullerian duct cyst _____

8. ligation of vas deferens _____

9. removal of foreign body, scrotum _____

10. I&D, abscess of epididymis _____

11. fixation of contralateral testis _____

12. incisional biopsy of testis followed by radical orchiectomy for tumor, inguinal approach _____

13. simple electrodesiccation of four lesions on penis _____

14. surgical excision of papilloma on penis, extensive procedure _____

15. spermatocele excision _____

16. spermatic vein ligation for varicocele, discontinued service _____

17. spermatic vein ligation for varicocele, laparoscopic surgery _____

18. clamp circumcision of newborn _____

19. corpora cavernosography with radiological S&I _____

20. deep penile I&D _____

21. Cecil repair, third stage _____

22. repair, hypospadias cripple _____

23. After undergoing a hypospadias repair 2 months ago, the patient injured his penis during a basketball game, and was operated on in order to repair it.

    _____

    _____

24. Patient presents with symptoms of deformity of his penis, and painful erection. The physician diagnosed Peyronie's disease and performed an injection and then excision of penile plaque.

    _____

    _____

25. Patient had suffered from frequent urination, pressure, and pain in the bladder. Upon examination, the physician found a prostate mass. Due to the size and specific location of the mass, an incisional biopsy of the prostate was performed to determine if the mass was benign or malignant.

    _____

    _____

NAME _____

# Female Genital System; Maternity Care and Delivery
## Codes 56405–59899

The codes in these surgical subsections of CPT cover procedures performed on the female genital system and for maternity care and delivery. In the female genital system, codes for body site and for in vitro fertilization are listed by the type of procedure.

The maternity care and delivery codes have a unique organization. They are grouped as follows: antepartum services; excision; introduction; repair; vaginal delivery, antepartum and postpartum care (normal uncomplicated cases); cesarean delivery; delivery after previous cesarean delivery; abortion; and other procedures.

## CODING TIP

### The Obstetric Package
The guidelines for maternity care/delivery describe the obstetric package of services normally provided for uncomplicated cases. The package consists of antepartum care, delivery, and postpartum care, as described. Before coding obstetrical services, study these notes carefully to avoid unbundling—improperly reporting work that is part of the package. Understanding the obstetric package also permits correct reporting of those services that are not part of the package and that can be coded separately.

## Provide codes for the following procedures. Include any necessary modifiers. In some cases, more than one code is required.

1. simple destruction of four lesions, vulva _____

2. complete radical vulvectomy _____

3. fitting and insertion of pessary _____

4. laser destruction of vaginal lesions (simple) _____

5. D&C, cervical stump _____

6. D&C, postpartum hemorrhage _____

7. uterine suspension _____

8. total abdominal hysterectomy _____

9. subtotal hysterectomy _____

CPT only © 2010 American Medical Association. All rights reserved.

10. insertion of IUD _____

11. routine obstetric care/vaginal delivery, previous cesarean delivery

    _____

12. miscarriage surgically completed in first trimester _____

13. abortion induced by D&C _____

14. cesarean delivery, surgical care only _____

15. cesarean delivery, including postpartum care, and total hysterectomy following attempted vaginal delivery; patient had previous cesarean delivery _____

16. Strassman type hysteroplasty and closure of vesicouterine fistula

    _____

17. chromotubation of oviduct including materials _____

18. laparoscopic assisted vaginal hysterectomy (uterus less than 250 grams)

    _____

19. multifetal pregnancy reductions _____

20. episiotomy by assisting physician _____

21. Making a small abdominal incision, the physician drains a cyst from each ovary. _____

22. An elderly woman without any prior history of cancer is diagnosed with an extensive malignant vaginal cancer, requiring vaginectomy and complete removal of the vaginal wall.

    _____

23. An obstetrician has been seeing this patient starting with her first visit to determine that she is pregnant. She recently performed the vaginal delivery, and the patient is now being seen in the office for her last postpartum visit. How will the obstetrician code for her services?

    _____

24. Patient has a hysterotomy to remove a hydatidiform mole as well as tubal ligation during the same surgical session.

    _____

25. A patient is pregnant with her fourth child and is having contractions that are rapidly coming closer together. She and her husband leave for the hospital, but the baby is born in the car before reaching the hospital. Once the baby is secured by emergency medical technicians, the patient is admitted and her physician delivers the placenta.

    _____

# Endocrine System; Nervous System

## Codes 60000–64999

The brief endocrine system subsection of the CPT Surgery Section contains codes for procedures on the thyroid gland, parathyroid, thymus, adrenal glands, and carotid body. The nervous system subsection comprises codes for nerves located in the skull, meninges, and brain; spine and spinal cord; extra-cranial nerves, peripheral nerves, and autonomic nervous system. Like the cardiovascular system section, the nervous system codes are complex, based on the particular anatomy and procedures required. Advances in techniques such as deep brain stimulation and pain management often lead to new and revised procedural codes in this section.

---

### CODING TIP

*Procedures Exempt from the -51 Modifier*

In addition to add-on procedures or services, there are other procedures in CPT with which a -51 modifier for multiple surgical procedures cannot be used. The -51 modifier identifies additional surgical procedures that are done during the major, or primary, surgery. The primary procedure is paid in full, and the additional procedures automatically receive reduced payment. Modifier -51 exempt codes are identified with the symbol ⊘.

---

## Provide codes for the following procedures. Include any necessary modifiers. In some cases, more than one code is required.

1. total thyroid lobectomy _____

2. twist drill hole for subdural puncture _____

3. resection of a vascular lesion at the base of the posterior cranial fossa

   _____

4. craniotomy for repair of dural/CSF leak _____

5. exploratory craniectomy _____

6. aspiration of thyroid cyst _____

7. laparoscopic adrenalectomy _____

8. parathyroidectomy _____

9. total thyroidectomy, limited neck dissection, for excision of malignancy

   _____

10. adrenalectomy _____

11. implantation of intrathecal drug infusion programmable pump _____

12. epidural percutaneous implantation of neurostimulator electrodes

    _____

13. implantation of cranial nerve neurostimulator electrodes

    _____

## Provide codes and decide whether to append the -51 modifier.

14. craniectomy, infratentorial, to excise a brain abscess, and twist drill

    hole to implant ventricular catheter _____

15. vertebral corpectomy with decompression of spinal cord, three

    segments _____

16. A 57-year-old patient who had suffered from muscular tremors due to Parkinson's disease was treated with an intracranial neurostimulator. She now needs to have the electrodes removed, and surgery is performed to remove them. _____

17. A young patient was born with hydrocephalus due to the accumulation of cerebrospinal fluid (CSF) in the ventricles of his brain. He is now scheduled for surgery to allow the neurosurgeon to create/implant a shunt that will drain the CSF into the peritoneum, thereby relieving the pressure on the brain. _____

18. After months of back pain, a patient is scheduled for an MRI scan of the spinal cord. The scan shows a lesion in the thoracic spine near T1 and T2. The physician performs a percutaneous needle biopsy of the spinal cord, using CT scan for the radiological supervision and interpretation of the needle placement. _____

19. The lamina of the lumbar spine at L3 and L4 are compressing the spinal cord, causing great pain. The surgeon explains that she will remove a portion of lamina at both segments to decompress the spinal cord, but there will be no removal of the vertebral facets, disks or foraminotomy. The surgeon had previously determined that the compression problem is not caused by spondylolisthesis. _____

20. The discovery of an intracranial abscess located above the tentorium and another below the tentorium leads to the performance of a craniectomy to drain each abscess. _____

# Eye and Ocular Adnexa; Auditory System; Operating Microscope

## Codes 65091–69990

Codes in these subsections of CPT's Surgery Section are used to report surgical procedures on the eye, its surrounding structures, and the ear. Ophthalmological diagnostic and treatment services are not coded from the Eye and Ocular Adnexa codes. Use the Ophthalmology codes in the Medicine Section instead.

---

### CODING TIP

*Operating Microscope*

An operating microscope—code 69990—is used in the performance of delicate surgical procedures. In some cases, CPT permits reporting of the operating microscope; in other cases, its use is always part of the procedure, and it cannot be reported in addition to the operation. For example, a note at the beginning of the eye and ocular adnexa subsection states that the operating microscope should not be reported in addition to codes 65091 to 68850—that is, with all the codes in this subsection. Be sure to review all notes when selecting codes.

---

**Provide codes for the following procedures. Include any necessary modifiers. In some cases, more than one code is required.**

1. removal of embedded foreign body, eyelid _____

2. biopsy, conjunctiva _____

3. ear piercing _____

4. removal, electromagnetic bone conduction hearing device, temporal bone _____

5. complete mastoidectomy _____

6. canthotomy _____

7. closure of eyelids by suture, temporary _____

8. scleral reinforcement without graft _____

9. extracapsular cataract removal with insertion of intraocular lens prothesis, mechanical technique _____

10. excision of scleral lesion _____

11. chalazion excision during the global period of a strabismus surgery

_____

12. tympanic membrane repair with operating microscope _____

13. biopsy of both external ears _____

14. impacted cerumen removed from both ears _____

15. ocular implant removal with operating microscope _____

16. removal of dislocated intracapsular lens _____

17. discontinued myringoplasty _____

18. biopsy and excision of exostoses from external auditory canal _____

19. tympanic neurectomy of both ears _____

20. canthus reconstruction, surgical care only _____

21. A 70-year-old patient with chronic glaucoma is still suffering from ele-
    vated intraocular pressure which has not responded to medical therapy.
    To treat the problem surgically, the surgeon will have to destroy por-
    tions of the ciliary body to bring down the intraocular pressure. The
    surgeon elects to do this with a freezing probe (cryotherapy) to destroy
    the ciliary process._____

22. This patient has been nearsighted all his adult life. Neither glasses nor
    contact lenses have sufficiently alleviated the problem, and the patient
    elects to have surgery. After applying topical anesthetic, the surgeon
    makes radial incisions on the anterior surface of the cornea, thereby
    flattening the cornea and correcting the refractive state. _____

23. A patient suddenly suffers from loss of vision in the right eye and goes
    to see the ophthalmologist. The examination shows that the retina of the
    right eye has detached and fallen into the posterior chamber of the eye
    causing loss of blood supply to the retina. The problem can be corrected
    with a retinal detachment repair by photocoagulation. The first repair is
    done the next day, and two more repairs are scheduled to be done within
    a 2-month treatment period. Code for the retinal detachment repairs.

    _____

24. The lacrimal sac, which is part of the lacrimal system that produces
    tears, has an abscess that must be drained in order for the lacrimal sys-
    tem to function properly. The surgeon makes a small incision directly
    into the lacrimal sac, and the pressure caused by the abscess is relieved
    as the area drains. The incision is sutured closed. _____

25. A senile elderly patient in a nursing home placed an earring in her ear
    which is now lodged in the external auditory canal. The patient's ten-
    dency to flail her arms whenever she is examined requires that general
    anesthesia be used to extract the earring. Once the patient has been
    anesthetized, the physician is able to visualize the earring and extract it
    with forceps and suction. _____

# Radiology Section

## Codes 70010–79999

The codes in the Radiology Section of CPT are used to report radiological services performed by or supervised by a physician, such as interpreting x-ray, ultrasound, and other types of imaging tests, and interventional radiology (image-guided surgery), in which diseases are treated nonoperatively using small catheters or other devices guided by radiological imaging. Codes in the diagnostic radiology and diagnostic ultrasound subsections are grouped anatomically. Radiation oncology and nuclear medicine subsection codes are arranged by service type.

Almost all radiology procedures have two parts: (1) a technical component, covering the technologist, the equipment, and processing, and (2) a professional component that includes the reading of the radiological examination and the physician's written interpretation report.

---

### CODING TIP

#### Unlisted Procedures and Special Reports

Because of advances in medical knowledge and techniques, a new procedure may not have a Category I or a Category III code. Such procedures are reported using "unlisted" codes in each section. The unlisted procedure codes, which always end in 99 (for example, 79999), are printed in the section guidelines and also appear at the ends of their code sections.

Advances are especially common in the area of radiology services with the introduction of newer, faster, and better imaging technology. CPT has codes for 16 unlisted code areas in radiology. When unlisted codes are reported, a special report must be attached that defines the nature of, extent of, and need for the procedure, and describes the time, effort, and equipment necessary to provide it.

---

**Provide radiology codes for the following procedures. Do not include the -26 modifier. In some cases, more than one code is required.**

1. radiologic examination of the ribs, two views (unilateral) _____

2. orthodontic cephalogram _____

3. magnetic resonance imaging of the pelvis (with contrast) _____

4. thoracic spine computerized tomography w/o contrast material _____

5. X-ray examination of the abdomen, single anteroposterior view _____

6. antegrade urography, S&I _____

7. serialographic thoracic aortography, S&I _____

8. complete study, cardiac MRI for function _____

9. bilateral external carotid angiography, S&I _____

10. unilateral adrenal angiography, S&I _____

11. CT bone density study and limited osseous survey _____

12. bilateral mammography _____

13. unlisted radiopharmaceutical therapeutic procedure _____

14. PET tumor imaging, whole body _____

15. SPECT myocardial imaging _____

16. diagnostic nuclear medicine procedure, gastrointestinal, unlisted

    _____

17. ten determinations of thyroid uptake _____

18. high-intensity brachytherapy, remote afterloading, 11 catheters _____

19. repeated Doppler echocardiography, fetal cardiovascular system _____

20. transluminal atherectomy, S&I, three peripheral arteries _____

21. To confirm the diagnosis of a rotator cuff tear, the physician first anes-
    thetizes the shoulder area and then, with a needle, injects contrast into
    the shoulder joint in order to visualize the area while taking a series of
    x-rays and interpreting what is found. Code for the physician's radio-
    logical supervision and interpretation of the x-rays. _____

22. After examination and testing by her internist, a young woman is still left
    with constant pelvic pain that cannot be diagnosed. The internist sends
    her for a CT scan with contrast to diagnose the problem. _____

23. An older construction worker developed eye pain after his sandblaster
    malfunctioned. He thought it was just "something in my eye," but after
    4 hours he was still in great pain and was seen by his ophthalmologist.
    The ophthalmologist examined the eye, but had difficulty determining
    what was in the eye due to an early cataract in the affected eye. The
    patient was sent for an ophthalmic ultrasound to find what foreign
    body was causing the problem. _____

24. One of the services provided by a radiation oncologist to patients who
    are receiving radiation therapy for cancer is clinical treatment planning.
    Code for the clinical treatment planning that encompasses a single
    treatment area in a single port with no blocking._____

25. A radiation oncologist reviews the port films, dosimetry, dose delivery,
    and treatment parameters, and also does a medical evaluation for a
    patient who receives eight treatments over 2 weeks. Code for the radia-
    tion oncologist's services related to the eight treatments. _____

# Pathology and Laboratory Section

## Codes 80047–89398

The codes in the Pathology and Laboratory Section of CPT cover services provided by physicians or by technicians under the supervision of physicians. These codes represent the services associated with performing the test and with analyzing and reporting the test results.

The codes are organized by the type of test: organ or disease oriented panels; drug testing; therapeutic drug assays; evocative/suppression testing; pathology consults; urinalysis; chemistry; hematology and coagulation; immunology; transfusion medicine; microbiology; anatomic pathology; cytopathology and cytogenetic studies; surgical pathology; and other procedures.

Note that since multiple procedures are commonly done on the same date of service, the -51 modifier is not used with codes from this section.

---

### CODING TIP

*Panels*

Individual tests that are customarily ordered together are grouped under laboratory panels. When a panel code is used, all the listed tests must have been performed. If not, the codes for the separate component tests that were done should be reported instead of a panel code. If a panel code is reported, no individual test within it may be additionally reported, but other tests outside it may be reported. Do not report panels with overlapping tests. In this case, report the panel with the greater number of performed tests, and report the other tests using individual test codes.

---

**Provide pathology and laboratory codes for the following procedures. Include any necessary modifiers. In some cases, more than one code is required. *Hint:* Check the required components of the organ/disease-oriented panels when coding multiple tests.**

1. total serum cholesterol _____

2. blood creatinine _____

3. 3-specimen GTT _____

4. FSH gonadotropin test _____

5. 2 hours, gastric secretory study _____

6. Saccomanno technique _____

7. hepatitis C, direct probe _____

8. commercial-kit urine culture _____

9. Rh blood typing _____

10. EA test for Epstein-Barr virus _____

11. urine specific gravity, automated, no microscopy _____

12. RPR, quantitative _____

13. potassium serum _____

14. HCG, quantitative _____

15. cholesterol, HDL, triglycerides, LDL _____

16. rubella screen _____

17. cryopreservation of five cell lines _____

18. HGH antibody _____

19. comprehensive clinical pathology consultation with report _____

20. mandated alcohol screen _____

21. A patient who had experienced chest pain and took a stress test has an abnormal reading. The cardiologist suspects a blockage in the coronary arteries and does a cardiac catheterization. This test shows the arteries are clear, but the aortic valve has an anomaly and has to be replaced. One of the tests the hospital will need both before and after surgery is the test that shows how long it takes for the blood to clot (bleeding time). Code for this test._____

22. After his most recent chemotherapy treatment, a patient was quite weakened. His oncologist ordered a complete CBC. _____

23. A patient with chronic edema despite years of treatment with diuretics is considered to have a pituitary gland problem that may be secreting excessive amounts of vasopressin, an antidiuretic hormone. Code for the ADH test._____

24. A patient presents with a 2-year history of urinary incontinence and pain when urinating. An examination shows an enlarge prostate gland, and his urologist now requests a test to check for the level of PSA, total.

    _____

25. A young woman with a family history of high cholesterol is now pregnant. Her obstetrician wants to do these lab studies to check her for both the routine obstetric blood work and a lipid profile:
    (a) Complete automated blood count and the appropriate manual differential WBC count, hepatitis B, rubella antibody, syphilis test, qualitative, RBC antibody screen, blood typing ABO and Rh(D).
    (b) Cholesterol serum total, lipoprotein, HDL cholesterol, triglycerides.
    Code the correct panels._____

# Medicine Section

## Codes 90281–99607

The Medicine Section of CPT contains the codes for the many types of evaluation, therapeutic, and diagnostic procedures that physicians perform. Most are considered noninvasive, in contrast to surgical procedures. The following major types of services are listed: immunizations, infusions, and chemotherapy; psychiatric; dialysis; gastroenterology; ophthalmology; cardiovascular; vascular and pulmonary studies; allergy and clinical immunology; neurology and neuromuscular; physical rehabilitation; and special services.

---

### CODING TIP

#### *Injections*

Injections and infusions of immune globulins, vaccines, toxoids, and other substances require two codes, one for administration and one for the particular vaccine or toxoid that is given. Chemotherapy and allergen immunotherapy, however, do not follow this guideline. The notes for each section should be observed. The AMA CPT website has the most recent new or revised vaccine product codes.

---

**Provide medicine codes for the following procedures. Include any necessary modifiers. In many cases, more than one code is required.**

1. subcutaneous injection of human rabies immune globulin _____

2. human immune globulin, intramuscular administration _____

3. intramuscular injection of Lyme disease vaccine _____

4. immunization with hepatitis A and hepatitis B vaccine _____

5. psychoanalysis _____

6. biofeedback training _____

7. hemodialysis procedure and single physician evaluation _____

8. diagnostic gastroenterology procedure, unlisted _____

9. fluorescein angiography _____

10. speech Stenger test _____

11. coronary thrombolysis by intracoronary infusion _____

12. limited transcranial Doppler study of intracranial arteries _____

13. total vital capacity _____

14. prick tests with allergenic extracts for (1) house dust, (2) seasonal

    grasses, (3) trees, (4) common ragweed, and (5) goldenrod _____

15. rapid desensitization procedure, discontinued _____

16. Preparation of chemotherapy agent followed by arterial infusion,

    3 hours _____

17. PUVA photochemotherapy _____

18. mandated occupational therapy reevaluation _____

19. IM injection of antibiotic _____

20. speech audiometry threshold test, one ear _____

# Medicine Section *continued*

## CODING TIP

### *Cardiac Catheterization*

Cardiac catheterizations are the most commonly performed surgical procedure. Complete coding of cardiac catheterization requires at least three codes: a code for the catheterization procedure itself, a code for the injection procedure, and a code for the imaging supervision and interpretation.

Be aware that cardiac catheterizations—the catheter insertion and the imaging supervision and interpretation services, not the injection procedure—each have a professional and a technical component. Unless the physician owns the laboratory, those codes are billed with the -26 modifier.

21. percutaneous transluminal pulmonary artery balloon angioplasty, three

    arteries _____

22. right heart catheterization in the hospital _____

23. catheter placement for coronary angiography, in physician-owned cath-

    eterization laboratory _____

24. unusually complicated and difficult combined right heart and retro-

    grade left heart catheterization _____

25. indicator dilution studies with arterial and venous catheterization, sub-

    sequent, in the hospital _____

26. percutaneous retrograde left heart catheterization from the femoral
    artery; injection procedure during the catheterization for aortography;
    and imaging supervision, interpretation, and report for aortography; in
    physician-owned cath laboratory

    _____

27. right heart catheterization and retrograde left heart catheterization for

    congenital anomalies, in the hospital _____

28. catheter placement in venous coronary bypass graft for coronary angi-
    ography; injection procedure for opacification of venous bypass graft;
    and imaging supervision, interpretation, and report; in physician-
    owned catheterization laboratory

    _____

29. The patient is seen for chest pain and shortness of breath. After months of medical treatment, the patient has a stress test with abnormal findings, a cardiac catheterization is performed, and a blockage is found in one of the coronary arteries. The surgeon explains that the blockage can be treated by percutaneous angioplasty, referred to as a PTCA, which involves the placement of a catheter through the skin into the affected artery, deploying a balloon that will remove the blockage. Code for the PTCA.

_____

_____

30. A newborn is not breathing correctly, and a congenital defect is suspected. Her physician recommends transthoracic echocardiography to determine the cause of the problem, because he suspects a malformation in the aortic valve and mitral valve.

_____

_____

31. Due to what may be an adverse reaction to longtime use of an antidepressant, a patient requires EEG monitoring for 2 hours to determine the brain's electrical activity. Sensors are placed on the patient's head to measure and record that activity. The physician then reviews the information and reports on his findings.

_____

_____

32. After allergy testing, a patient is diagnosed with allergies to bee and hornet stings. She is sent to an allergy specialist who prepares the allergenic extract for injection into the patient. The specialist also provides the single injection of the two stinging insect venoms.

_____

_____

33. A mother brings her child in to the pediatrician's office for a well visit. She knows that today her child will be getting the vaccine for DTP and MMR. Each vaccine will be given via separate injections. Code for the injections.

_____

_____

# Category II Codes

## Codes 0001F–7025F

The Category II code set contains supplemental tracking codes to help collect data regarding services, such as prenatal care and tobacco use cessation counseling, that are known to contribute to good patient care. Having codes available reduces the amount of administrative time needed to gather these data from documentation.

The use of these codes is optional and does not affect reimbursement. These codes are, however, used for pay-for-performance reporting, such as the PQRI program under CMS, in which case a bonus payment may result. The codes are not required for correct coding and are not a substitute for Category I codes.

Category II codes have an alphabetical character as the fifth character following the four digits in the code. They are arranged according to the following categories:

- Composite Measures
- Patient Management
- Patient History
- Physical Examination
- Diagnostic Screening Processes or Results
- Therapeutic, Preventive or Other Interventions
- Follow-Up or Other Outcomes
- Patient Safety

---

## CODING TIP

### Category II Code Updates

Category II codes are released twice a year: January 1 and July 1. The current listing and its effective date are available on the Internet at www.ama-assn.org/go/CPT.

---

## Provide the Category II codes for the following performance measures.

1. tobacco use cessation intervention, counseling _____

2. tobacco use, smoking, assessed _____

3. subsequent prenatal care visit _____

4. blood pressure, measured _____

5. postpartum care visit _____

# Category III Codes
## Codes 0019T–0259T

The Category III code set contains temporary codes for emerging technology, services, and procedures. If a Category III code is available for a new procedure, this code must be reported instead of a Category I unlisted code.

The codes in this section are not like CPT Category I codes, which require that the service/procedure be performed by many health care professionals in clinical practice in multiple locations and that FDA approval, as appropriate, has already been received. For these reasons, temporary codes for emerging technology, services, and procedures have been placed in a separate section of the CPT book. When a temporary service or procedure does meet these requirements, it is then listed as a Category I code in the appropriate section of the main text.

Category III codes have an alphabetical character as the fifth character following the four digits in the code.

## CODING TIP

### Category III Code Updates

Category III codes are released twice a year: January 1 and July 1. The current listing and its effective date are available on the Internet at www.ama-assn.org/go/CPT.

## Provide the Category III codes for the following.

1. insertion of a temporary prosthetic urethral stent _____

2. CT colonography; screening _____

3. speculoscopy exhaled breath condensate pH _____

4. Procalcitonin (PCT) _____

5. breath test for heart transplant rejection _____

6. high-dose rate electronic brachytherapy, per fraction _____

7. destruction of macular drusen, photocoagulation _____

8. insertion of anterior segment aqueous drainage device, without extra-ocular reservoir; internal approach _____

9. cerebral perfusion analysis using computed tomography with contrast administration _____

10. endovascular repair of abdominal aortic aneurysm, abdominal aorta involving visceral vessel, using fenestrated modular bifurcated prosthesis _____

# Health Care Common Procedure Coding System (HCPCS)

The Health Care Common Procedure Coding System (HCPCS) is used to report procedures and services not covered in CPT. HCPCS Level II is a HIPAA-mandated code set that is revised annually by CMS. New codes are effective January 1 of the year and must be used for services provided on or after that date.

Level II is made up of more than 2400 five-digit alphanumeric codes for items that are not listed in CPT. Most of these items are supplies, materials, or injections that may be covered by Medicare. For example, a HCPCS code from the J series of the Level II codes is used for the material (drug) that is injected, rather than a CPT code. Some items are new services or procedures that are not covered in CPT. Level II codes start with a letter followed by four digits, such as J7630. There are 22 sections, each covering a related group of items:

Transportation services
Medical and surgical supplies
Miscellaneous and experimental
Enteral and parenteral therapy
Temporary hospital outpatient PPS
Dental procedures
Durable medical equipment (DME)
Procedures and services, temporary
Rehabilitative services
Drugs administered other than oral method
Chemotherapy drugs
Temporary codes for DMERCS*
Orthotic procedures
Prosthetic procedures
Medical services
Pathology and laboratory
Temporary codes
Diagnostic radiology services
Private payer codes
State Medicaid agency codes
Vision and hearing services

---

*DMERC = Durable Medical Equipment Regional Carriers

The two-letter HCPCS modifiers are useful indicators of factors other than those covered by CPT modifiers. For example, there are HCPCS modifiers for each finger and each toe. The modifiers are to be used with both Level I and Level II codes.

HCPCS Level II codes and modifiers are available both from government sources and from many commercial publishers. Visit the CMS website for general HCPCS information at:

www.cms.gov/medhcpcsgeninfo/

---

## CODING TIP

### Locating Correct HCPCS Codes

The steps for locating correct codes using HCPCS Level II codes and modifiers are similar to those for CPT codes. First, locate the main term in the index, and then check the section listings to verify accuracy. Similar format rules also apply. Descriptors before a semicolon are common; the entries after it provide unique endings to complete the procedure. Note, however, that unlike CPT, many codes are differentiated by quantities or dosages. Check also for the need for modifiers.

---

## CODING TIP

### ABN Modifiers

HCPCS modifiers are used as CPT modifiers are used. For example, HCPCS modifiers distinguish between voluntary and required use of advanced beneficiary notices of noncoverage (ABNs):

-GA  Waiver of Liability Statement Issued, as Required by Payer Policy

-GX  Notice of Liability Issued, Voluntary under Payer Policy

-GK  Reasonable and Necessary Item or Service

-GY  Item/Service Statutorily Excluded

-GZ  Item/Service Expected to Be Denied as Not Reasonable and Necessary

---

# HCPCS Level II National Codes and Modifiers

**Provide HCPCS codes and modifiers for the following procedures.**

1.  standard wheelchair _____

2.  adjustable semirigid cervical molded chin cup _____

3.  WHFO with inflatable air chamber _____

4.  12-volt Utah battery and battery charger _____

5.  cardiokymography _____

6.  nonemergency BLS ambulance service _____

7.  nasal cannula _____

8.  occult blood test strips, for dialysis 100 _____

9.  drainable ostomy pouch with attached barrier _____

10. Levine type stomach tube _____

11. dysphagia screening _____

12. hearing aid fitting _____

13. anterior chamber intraocular lens _____

14. scratch resistant coating for a pair of glasses _____

15. static finger splint _____

16. 2 mg, dactinomycin _____

17. inhalation solution of beclomethasone, per milligram, DME administration, unit dose _____

18. isoetharine hydrochloride inhalation solution, DME administration, unit dose form, 1 milligram _____

19. administration, influenza virus vaccine _____

20. multiple PET myocardial perfusion imaging following rest ECG

    _____

21. hemodialysis machine _____

22. electric hospital bed with mattress _____

23. pickup folding walker, new _____

24. nonsegmental home model, pneumatic compressor, rental _____

25. one gram of wound filler hydrocolloid dressing, dry form _____

## For the following, supply the CPT (HCPCS Level I) code or codes, as well as HCPCS modifiers, if appropriate.

26. excision of 1.0 cm benign lesion from upper right eyelid _____

27. release of thenar muscle, left thumb _____

28. acute chiropractic manipulative treatment, one spinal region _____

29. anesthesia for closed procedure in hip joint personally performed by anesthesiologist _____

30. ligation of anomalous left anterior descending coronary artery

_____

31. hallux valgus correction, left foot, great toe _____

32. single determination, noninvasive pulse oximetry for oxygen saturation, technical component _____

33. extracapsular cataract extraction and insertion of IOL, performed in ambulatory surgical center _____

34. automated dip stick urinalysis, CLIA-waived test _____

35. closed treatment of acetabulum fracture with manipulation, right hip

_____

# Coding Quiz: CPT and HCPCS

NAME _____

_____ 1. A cardiovascular surgeon begins to perform a percutaneous transcatheter placement of an intracoronary stent, but stops the procedure because of the patient's respiratory distress. Select the correct code.

&#9312; 92982
&#9313; 92980
&#9314; 92980-52
&#9315; 92980-53

_____ 2. A metal splinter was removed from the posterior segment of both eyes' ocular area using a magnet. Choose the correct code.

&#9312; 65260-52
&#9313; 65260-50
&#9314; 65235
&#9315; 65265

_____ 3. A surgeon performs a diagnostic ERCP and a trocar bladder aspiration. Which codes are correct?

&#9312; 43260, 51005-22
&#9313; 43260, 51005-51
&#9314; 43260, 51101-59
&#9315; 43260, 51005-62

_____ 4. A patient has an office encounter for removal of five skin tags on her hand. During the visit, she asks the physician to evaluate swelling and heat in her left knee. The physician performs an expanded history and examination with low medical decision making. What codes should be reported?

&#9312; 11200, 99214
&#9313; 11200, 99213-25
&#9314; 11100, 99213-25
&#9315; 11200, 99213-51

_____ 5. Following surgery to repair a sliding inguinal hernia, the patient is turned over to his primary care physician for all follow-up care. Which is the correct code for that follow-up care?

&#9312; 49525-55
&#9313; 49525-25
&#9314; 49525-77
&#9315; 49525-24

_____ 6. What is the correct code for a home visit with an established patient that required a detailed history of what has occurred since the physician's previous visit, a detailed examination, and moderately complex medical decision making?

    ① 99243
    ② 99343
    ③ 99349
    ④ 99313

_____ 7. A patient is referred to a specialist, who performs an E/M service in the office and prepares a written report for the referring physician. From what code range is the correct code chosen?

    ① 99241–99245
    ② 99251–99255
    ③ 99261–99263
    ④ 99271–99275

_____ 8. Selecting a code from the range for emergency department services depends on:

    ① whether the patient is new or established
    ② whether the patient is new or established, and what type of history is taken
    ③ the type of history, examination, and medical decision making performed
    ④ the type of history/examination performed and the amount of time spent

_____ 9. The physician is asked by the patient to perform a cardiovascular health risk assessment to evaluate his probability for heart disease. Which code is correct?

    ① 99401
    ② 99401-22
    ③ 99272
    ④ 99420

_____ 10. Modifier -47 is used for anesthesia services performed under difficult circumstances.

    ① True
    ② False

_____ 11. Which set of codes correctly describes the anesthesia services for insertion of a cardioverter/defibrillator via a transthoracic approach in a patient with severe systemic disease?

    ① 00534-P3
    ② 00560-P3
    ③ 00534-P4
    ④ 00560-P4

_____ 12. The correct code for a postoperative visit for the purpose of documentation is:

① 99070
② 99025
③ 99024
④ 99217

_____ 13. A global surgery code for a diagnostic procedure includes follow-up care related only to recovery from the procedure itself, not for care of the patient's underlying condition.

① True
② False

_____ 14. A patient's 3.9-cm benign lesion excision on the arm is followed by an intermediate repair involving a layered closure of 4.5 cm. Select the correct code(s).

① 11404
② 12002, 11424-51
③ 12002, 11404-51
④ 12032, 11404-51

_____ 15. A surgeon applied a 200 sq cm xenograft. The correct code(s) are:

① 15400, 15401-51
② 15400, 15401
③ 15350, 15351-58
④ 15050

_____ 16. A surgeon excised a chest wall tumor involving the ribs and then performed a mediastinal lymphadenectomy, followed by plastic reconstruction. Select the correct code(s).

① 19301, 19302-51
② 19260, 19272
③ 19272
④ 19301, 19272-51

_____ 17. After initiating a regional Bier block, a surgeon performs a closed treatment of an ulnar shaft fracture; the surgeon monitored the patient and the block during the surgery. Select the correct code(s) for this service.

① 25530, 01820-47
② 25530-47
③ 25530
④ 01820, 25530

_____ 18. Following the open treatment of a fractured big toe, the surgeon applies an ambulatory-type short leg cast. Choose the correct code(s).

    ① 28515
    ② 28525
    ③ 28505
    ④ 28505, 29425

_____ 19. A patient had a previous operation 15 days ago to treat a dislocated ankle. Today, the same surgeon repairs the patient's flexor tendon on the other foot. What code should be reported for today's service?

    ① 28200-79
    ② 28200
    ③ 28200-58
    ④ 28200-51

_____ 20. A physician removes a foreign body from a patient's nose during an office visit; local anesthesia was required. Should the anesthesia administration be reported for reimbursement?

    ① Yes
    ② No

_____ 21. Diagnostic endoscopy is performed on the left nasal cavity. Select the correct code.

    ① 31237
    ② 31231-52
    ③ 31231-50
    ④ 31231

_____ 22. Select the correct code(s) for a segmentectomy and bronchoplasty.

    ① 32484, 32501-51
    ② 32484, 32501
    ③ 32484, 31770-51
    ④ 32501

_____ 23. A cardiologist performs a second pericardiocentesis and provides supervision/interpretation of the radiological procedures. Choose the correct code(s).

    ① 33010
    ② 33010-26
    ③ 33011, 76930
    ④ 33011, 76930-26

_____ 24. Combined arterial and venous grafting for a coronary bypass is coded using the range 33517–33523.

    ① True
    ② False

_____ 25. The repair of a ruptured aneurysm of the abdominal aorta is made extremely complicated by the patient's obesity; the procedure takes twice as long as normally anticipated, which is appropriately documented in the operative report. Select the correct code.

① 35001
② 35082-21
③ 35082
④ 35082-22

_____ 26. Following a diagnostic thoracoscopy and biopsy of the mediastinal space, the surgeon performs a surgical thorascopy and excises a mediastinal mass. Select the correct code(s).

① 32606, 32662-51
② 32606, 32662-59
③ 32662
④ 32601, 32606

_____ 27. The correct reporting of a separate procedure that is not done as part of a surgical package requires which of the following modifiers?

① -51
② -54
③ -59
④ -99

_____ 28. The correct code for a laparoscopically aided esophagogastric fundo-plasty is 43280. What is the code for the same procedure using an open approach?

① 43289
② 43324
③ 43325
④ 49320

_____ 29. A surgeon performs a modified radical mastectomy, including the axillary lymph nodes, following an incisional breast biopsy which results in a finding of malignancy. Select the correct code(s) for these procedures.

① 19240, 19101
② 19240, 19101-51
③ 19307
④ 19240-52

_____ 30. A cesarean delivery followed an attempted vaginal delivery. The mother's previous children had been born with cesarean delivery. The physician handled both the delivery and routine antepartum and postpartum care. Select the correct code.

① 59618
② 59620
③ 59622
④ 59610

_____ 31. The surgeon created a twist drill hole for subdural puncture in order to implant a pressure recording device. Select the correct code(s).

① 61105, 61107-51
② 61105, 61107-59
③ 61105, 61107
④ 61107

_____ 32. Many radiology procedures have two parts:

① unlisted or guided
② supervision or interpretation
③ professional or technical
④ complete or partial

_____ 33. The correct code for the supervision and interpretation of a selective, unilateral angiography of an external carotid artery is:

① 75660-26
② 75662-26
③ 75660
④ 75662

_____ 34. Select the correct code(s) for these laboratory tests: carbon dioxide, sodium, urea nitrogen, creatinine, chloride, calcium, glucose, and potassium.

① 82374, 84295, 84520, 82565, 82435, 82310, 82947, 84132
② 80051, 82310, 82565, 84520
③ 80053
④ 80048

_____ 35. A growth hormone stimulation panel and an aldosterone test are ordered. Choose the correct code(s).

① 80428, 82088-51
② 80428, 82088
③ 80428, 82088-59
④ 80435, 82088

_____ 36. An intravenous injection of immune globulin, 1 g, is administered to a Medicare patient. Choose the correct code(s).

① 90283, 90784
② 90281, 90782
③ J1561, 96374
④ J1561

_____ 37. A cardiologist performed a percutaneous retrograde left heart cardiac catheterization from the femoral artery requiring left atrial angiography. The cardiologist provided imaging supervision, interpretation, and report. Select the correct codes.

    ① 93511, 93542, 93561
    ② 93542, 93555
    ③ 93510, 93543, 93555-26
    ④ 93510, 93543, 93556

_____ 38. To study a patient's sleep disorder, a neurologist conducted an extended 4-hour monitoring of the patient's EEG. Choose the correct code.

    ① 95812
    ② 95813
    ③ 95813-22
    ④ 95816

_____ 39. For a Medicare patient, which range of codes is used for prosthetic procedures?

    ① L5000–L8699
    ② M0064–M0302
    ③ J0120–J8999
    ④ A4206–A6406

_____ 40. A Medicare patient is prescribed a wheelchair with detachable arms and leg rests. Which code is correct?

    ① E1050
    ② E1083
    ③ E1150
    ④ E1160

# *Part* 3 Physician and Facility Coding Linkage and Compliance

Under the regulations of HIPAA, providers are required to use multiple coding systems to code single episodes in order to satisfy the data needs for reimbursement, case mix analysis, practice profiling, research, and outcomes measurement. The illustration on the next page reviews the basic steps in the medical coding process and the code sets that are required for the various billing settings.

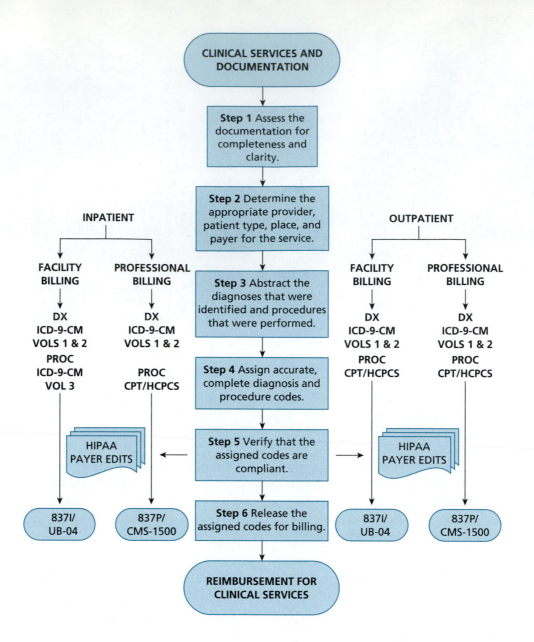

*Facility (institutional) billing* refers to charging payers and patients for the costs incurred by the hospital or other entity in the delivery of health care. *Professional billing,* on the other hand, refers to charging for the costs of providing physicians' or other professional providers' services, such as those of a surgeon, a nurse practitioner, or a CRNA. When the physician provides services, treatments, and procedures in the physician's office or other physician-owned setting, the physician's charges incorporate the cost of the "facility." When the physician performs professional work in the hospital, however, the physician is charging for the particular procedures, and the hospital is charging for the facility's part of the costs, such as:

- Room and board
- Medications
- Ancillary tests and procedures

- Equipment/supplied used during surgery or therapy
- The amount of time spent in an operating room, recovery room, or intensive care unit
- Administrative and patient care services

In the *inpatient* setting, for *facility billing*, the medical coder in the Health Information Management (HIM) department assigns both diagnosis and procedure codes based on the ICD-9-CM. Volumes 1 and 2 are used to classify the diagnoses. The principal diagnosis (Pdx)—the condition established after study as the chief reason for the patient's admission—is listed first, followed by other, secondary diagnosis codes. Volume 3 is the source for inpatient procedure codes, which result in reimbursement to the facility for all the services it provided.

In the *inpatient* setting, for *professional billing*, the medical coder who is employed by the physician practice assigns diagnosis codes based on ICD-9-CM and procedure codes based on CPT/HCPCS.

In the *outpatient* setting, for both *facility and professional billing*, the medical coder assigns diagnosis codes again based on volumes 1 and 2 of the ICD-9-CM. Procedures are coded using the CPT/HCPCS code set.

# Code Linkage

On correct claims, each reported service is connected to a diagnosis that supports the necessity of the procedure to investigate or treat the patient's condition. This connection between the diagnostic and the procedural information, called *code linkage*, establishes the medical necessity—medical services' baseline—of the reported charges. Correct claims also comply with the many other requirements issued by government and private payers, such as those dealing with the place, frequency, and/or level of services or specific documentation.

To establish medical necessity, the payer must understand the patient's condition—how severe it is, or how it is emerging—and everything about signs, symptoms, or history that relates to the reason for care. These facts must be documented in the patient's medical record as well as in the codes.

Claims are denied due to lack of medical necessity when the reported services are not consistent with the symptoms or the diagnosis, or are not in keeping with generally accepted professional medical standards. Correctly linked codes that support medical necessity meet these conditions:

- The CPT procedure codes match the ICD-9-CM diagnosis codes.
- The procedures are not elective, experimental, or nonessential.
- The procedures are furnished at an appropriate level.

Medical necessity edits are established by each third-party payer. For example, Medicare carriers have their own rules for particular procedures and the diagnoses that must be linked for payment. Private payers may impose different edits.

# Common Coding Errors

All codes must be currently correct and complete. Errors include:

- Truncated coding—diagnosis codes are not reported at the highest level of specificity available
- Out-of-date codes

- Assumption coding—reporting items or services that are not actually documented, but that the coder assumes were performed
- Altering documentation after the services are reported
- Coding without proper documentation
- Reporting services provided by unlicensed or unqualified clinical personnel
- Failing to have all necessary documentation available at the time of coding
- Failing to satisfy the conditions of coverage for a particular service, such as the physician's direct supervision of a radiology technician's work
- Failing to comply with the unique billing requirements for a particular service, such as the rules for global surgical period coverage
- Reporting services that are not covered or that have limited coverage
- Using modifiers incorrectly, or not at all
- Upcoding—using a procedure code that provides a higher reimbursement rate than the code that actually reflects the service provided
- Unbundling—billing the parts of a bundled procedure as separate procedures

# Coding Compliance

The *Medical Coding Workbook for Physician Practices and Facilities* is designed to build your skill in accurately linking diagnosis and procedure codes and correctly reporting them. Each set of exercises begins with a *Coding Tip* that explains an important rule concerning linkage and compliance. After completion of all the exercises in this part, you will know how to apply these guidelines:

- Verifying linkage
- Selecting the primary condition
- Reporting chronic or undiagnosed conditions
- Using V and E codes for a clear picture of an encounter
- Avoiding unspecified diagnosis codes
- Reporting complications
- Reporting global procedures and laboratory panels
- Using correct code sets
- Following the *ICD-9-CM Official Guidelines for Coding and Reporting*

NAME _____

# Section 1

The following diagnosis and procedure codes have been reported. In each case, indicate whether the codes are correctly linked ("Y" for yes) or not correctly linked ("N" for no).

| ICD-9-CM | CPT | Linked? |
| --- | --- | --- |
| 1. 692.71 | 99201 | _____ |
| 2. 410.01 | 99223 | _____ |
| 3. 599.70, 788.41, 789.07 | 50600 | _____ |
| 4. 216.1 | 67961 | _____ |
| 5. 560.1 | 27147 | _____ |
| 6. 766.2 | 99382 | _____ |
| 7. 754.0 | 30520 | _____ |
| 8. 250.51, 362.02 | 92012 | _____ |
| 9. 733.81, 905.2 | 27824 | _____ |
| 10. 568.0 | 56810 | _____ |

NAME _____

# Section 2

## CODING TIP

### *Selecting the Primary Diagnosis*

The primary diagnosis, or condition, is the most important reason for the care provided. It is reported first, if more than one condition is pertinent or treated. Additional codes are listed to describe all documented, current coexisting conditions that affect patient treatment or require treatment during the encounter. Coexisting conditions may be related to the primary diagnosis, or they may involve a separate illness that the physician diagnoses and treats during the encounter. Only the definitive condition or conditions that caused the encounter are coded. Symptoms that are integral to a diagnosis, such as stomach pain related to bowel obstruction, are not reported.

Some conditions require the assignment of two codes. A code may be needed for the disease's etiology and another for its manifestation, or typical signs or symptoms. Manifestation codes are shown in italics in the ICD-9-CM and are never primary, even when the diagnostic statement is written in that order. In some cases, a combination code may cover both etiology and manifestation.

**Provide the diagnosis codes for the following statements. If sufficient information is given, also provide the procedure code. List the ICD-9-CM codes in the correct order, followed by the CPT codes.**

1. severe abdominal pain, nausea, and vomiting from acute pancreatitis

   _____

2. vitamin B deficiency and sideroblastic anemia

   _____

3. cerebellar ataxia and hepatitis in chronic episodic alcoholism

   _____

4. pneumonia due to parainfluenza virus; radiologic examination of chest, special views

   _____

5. generalized peritonitis and acute appendicitis; appendectomy for ruptured appendix

   _____

6. direct ligation of esophageal varices due to portal hypertension

   _____

7. patient complained of hematuria and pyuria; urinalysis by bacterial culture of urine by commercial kit confirms acute pyelonephritis due to E. coli infection

   _____

8. physician performs cystourethroscopy with bilateral meatotomy to remove a foreign body in the genitourinary tract

   _____

9. postsurgical hypoglycemia and malnutrition; a breath hydrogen test is performed

   _____

10. due to dysmenorrhea and uterine endometriosis, physician performs a laparoscopic assisted vaginal hysterectomy, uterus less than 250 grams

   _____

# Section 3

## CODING TIP

### *Reporting Chronic or Undiagnosed Conditions*

A chronic condition—one that continues over a long period of time or recurs frequently—is reported each time the patient receives care for that condition. However, conditions that are no longer being treated or no longer exist are not reported, unless the documentation shows that a previous history is pertinent to the current condition. Some encounters cover both an acute and a chronic condition. If both the acute and the chronic illnesses are treated and each has a code, list the acute code first. Diagnoses are not always established at the first encounter. In this case, diagnosis codes that cover symptoms, signs, and ill-defined conditions are used. Inconclusive diagnoses, such as those preceded by "rule out," "suspected," or "probable," are not coded. Code only to the highest degree of certainty, listing the most definitive diagnosis first.

**Provide the diagnosis codes for the following statements. If sufficient information is given, also provide the procedure code. List the ICD-9-CM codes in the correct order, followed by the CPT codes.**

1. chronic and subacute arthropathy

   _____

2. encounter for chronic pleurisy with influenza

   _____

3. patient complains of blood in urine, frequent urination, and generalized abdominal pain; a tumor is suspected, and a diagnostic cystoscopy is scheduled

   _____

4. acute and chronic mesenteric lymphadenitis

   _____

5. vertigo; TIA suspected

   _____

6. pelvis swelling, probable malignant tumor

   _____

7. stereotactic needle core breast biopsy; finding of malignant primary
   tumor in upper-outer quadrant of left breast

   _____

8. routine 12-lead ECG with interpretation/report, abnormal finding

   _____

9. patient with chronic and acute maxillary sinusitis undergoes surgical
   nasal/sinus endoscopy and maxillary antrostomy

   _____

10. office consultation (comprehensive history and examination, moder-
    ately complex medical decision making) to evaluate complaints of
    nervousness, loss of sleep, and heat intolerance; diagnosis of thyrotoxi-
    cosis, rule out Graves' disease

    _____

NAME _____

# Section 4

---

### CODING TIP

*Using V and E Codes for a Clear Picture of an Encounter*

V codes, for factors influencing health status and contact with health services, and E codes, for external causes of injury and poisoning, are often required to provide a complete picture of the medical necessity for reported procedures. These codes may also help establish liability among payers, such as primary medical insurance and workers' compensation coverage.

Some V codes, such as those for general medical examinations and screening tests, are used as primary diagnoses. Others, such as V codes for a family or personal history of a disease, may not be used as primary; rather, they are listed as secondary codes. E codes are always secondary to the primary diagnosis, because their purpose is to describe a cause, not a condition or a reason for an encounter.

---

**Provide the diagnosis codes for the following statements. If sufficient information is given, also provide the procedure code. List the ICD-9-CM codes in the correct order, followed by the CPT codes.**

1. single assay HIV-1 and HIV-2 screening test for AIDS; patient has no HIV-related symptoms

   _____

2. intramuscular injection of hepatitis B globulin

   _____

3. annual medical examination of a 49-year-old male who is a new patient

   _____

4. bilateral screening mammography of patient whose mother and sister were diagnosed with breast cancer

   _____

5. normal vaginal delivery, antepartum/postpartum care, delivery of healthy boy

   _____

CPT only © 2010 American Medical Association. All rights reserved.

6. patient is a house painter who fell from scaffolding on the job and required closed treatment and manipulation of a humeral shaft fracture

   _____

7. local treatment of first-degree burns on both legs of an adult after clothing was burned by a bonfire

   _____

8. gastric intubation to remove stomach contents after patient was unconscious due to an accidental poisoning by an overdose of mescaline *Hint:* The diagnosis requires three codes—poisoning, manifestation, and cause.

   _____

9. office encounter with an established patient (expanded history/examination, low decision-making complexity) who has nausea and vomiting due to an adverse reaction to an antibiotic

   _____

10. surgical exploration of a complicated chest wound caused by shotgun accident

    _____

# Section 5

**For each of the following diagnostic statements, what information is missing that would permit the assignment of a specific ICD-9-CM code?**

1. patient complains of abdominal pain

   _____

   _____

2. gastric or intestinal hemorrhage

   _____

   _____

3. chronic bronchitis

   _____

   _____

4. acute myocardial infarction, location specified

   _____

   _____

5. chronic suppurative otitis media

   _____

   _____

6. acute reaction to stress

_____

_____

7. diabetes mellitus

_____

_____

8. monocytic leukemia in remission

_____

_____

9. streptococcus infection

_____

_____

10. osteoarthrosis

_____

_____

# Section 6

## CODING TIP

### *Reporting Surgical Diagnoses and Complications*

When surgery is performed and the preoperative diagnosis changes, the new postoperative diagnosis code is reported, rather than the preoperative code.

If complications arise during the procedure, the primary diagnosis is the first code reported. The complication is coded in addition, following the primary diagnosis. However, if the complications arise after the procedure is complete and require an additional procedure, the complication is the primary diagnosis for the later procedure. Many complications of surgical and medical care are contained in categories 996–999.

**Provide the diagnosis codes for the following statements. If sufficient information is given, also provide the procedure code. List the ICD-9-CM codes in the correct order, followed by the CPT codes. *Hint:* Some procedures require the use of a modifier.**

1. mechanical complication due to automatic implantable cardiac defibrillator

   _____

2. accidental puncture of the stomach during surgery

   _____

3. septicemia after repair of an open wound

   _____

4. vaccinia resulting from an immunization

   _____

5. complications arising after an incompatible blood transfusion

   _____

6. *Staphylococcus aureus* septicemia due to an indwelling urinary catheter

   _____

7. during a procedure to implant a patient-activated cardiac event recorder, a hemorrhage occurs

   _____

8. 12 hours following surgery for an acute myocardial infarction, the electrode of a cardiac pacemaker fails, requiring additional surgery

   _____

9. following removal of a 2.5-cm tumor from the trunk of a patient, the pathology report indicates that it is malignant

   _____

10. a laparoscopic cholecystectomy is performed for a patient with acute cholecystitis; during the procedure, the patient has cardiac arrest, and after reviving the patient, the surgeon terminates the procedure

    _____

# Section 7

---

## CODING TIP

### *Reporting Bundled (Global) Procedures and Laboratory Panels*

Unbundling—reporting procedures that are covered under another code as additional work—of surgical codes and of laboratory panels is non-compliant. A careful reading of the section notes and procedural descriptors in CPT indicates which procedures are included in various codes.

General principles also apply. For example, surgical procedures always include the diagnostic procedures that precede them (on the same day of service). An application of this point is the fact that when a biopsy precedes the excision of a lesion, only the excision is reported.

It is also important to review the individual tests that comprise each laboratory panel. Multiple panels are often ordered. If the component tests overlap, only one panel is reported, along with the differing individual tests from the other panels.

---

## CODING TIP

### *Using Correct Code Sets*

Use of the proper code set, such as HCPCS codes as applicable for supplies, must also be double-checked.

---

### Provide both the diagnostic and procedure codes for the following statements.

1. During an annual physical examination of a 62-year-old female established patient with a family history of kidney disease, the physician orders a comprehensive metabolic panel and a renal function panel.

   _____

2. Patient has blood in stool; physician performs a diagnostic sigmoidoscopy followed by removal of a foreign body.

   _____

3.  Patient has a closed fracture of the tibial shaft; physician performs a closed treatment and applies an ambulatory short leg cast.

    _____

4.  Following a biopsy, two benign sebaceous cystic skin lesions are excised—a 4.2-cm lesion from the hand of the patient and a 3.3-cm lesion from the patient's back; surgeon administered local anesthesia.

    _____

5.  Patient has suffered an open fracture of multiple sites of her lower jaw bone when the car in which she was a passenger hit the highway divider; surgeon performs an open treatment that requires multiple approaches, including internal fixation, interdental fixation, and wiring of dentures.

    _____

6.  Physician performs an endoscopically aided diagnostic bronchoscopy and a transbronchial lung biopsy under fluoroscopic guidance for a patient with pneumonia due to adenovirus.

    _____

7.  Physician orders laboratory tests of total serum cholesterol, direct measurement of HDL cholesterol, and triglycerides for a patient with essential hypertension.

    _____

8.  Elderly patient has been diagnosed with a mature cataract in the left eye; surgeon performs a one-stage extracapsular cataract removal with iridectomy, use of viscoelastic agents, and subconjunctival injections, and then inserts an intraocular lens prosthesis.

    _____

9.  Patient has been diagnosed with carcinoma in situ of the prostate; surgeon performs a complete transurethral electrosurgical resection of the prostate; the procedure includes a vasectomy, meatotomy, cystourethroscopy, urethral calibration, and internal urethrotomy; control of postoperative bleeding is also required.

    _____

10. After a comprehensive ophthalmological examination of a new Medicare patient, the ophthalmologist prescribes a corneal lens for the left eye; supplying the bifocal gas permeable contact lens is also reported.

    _____

NAME _____

# Section 8

## CODING TIP

### ICD-9-CM Official Guidelines for Coding and Reporting

Both inpatient and outpatient (physician practice) coding must follow the ICD-9-CM Official Guidelines for Coding and Reporting, which has these sections: I. Conventions, General Coding Guidelines, and Chapter-Specific Guidelines; II. Selection of Principal Diagnosis; III. Reporting Additional Diagnoses; IV. Diagnostic Coding and Reporting Guidelines for Outpatient Services; and Appendix I. Present on Admission Reporting Guidelines. The current guidelines are available at www.cdc.gov/nchs/icd/icd9cm_addenda_guidelines.htm.

## CODING TIP

### ICD-9-CM Volume 3

The third volume of ICD-9-CM is mandated for use in reporting inpatient procedures, treatments, and services. Codes are researched in the standard way by locating the key term in the Index to Procedures and then verifying the code in the Tabular Listing of procedures. Note that on October 1, 2013, a transition to the ICD-10-PCS code set will be mandated.

## A. Provide the diagnostic codes for the following statements.

1. Patient presents to the hospital with nausea and vomiting 4 hours after receiving chemotherapy for acute lymphocytic leukemia. She is readmitted for IV fluids and antiemetics. It is determined the nausea and vomiting are due to the chemotherapy.

   Principal/Other Diagnoses_____

2. Patient presents to the emergency room complaining of dizziness and headache postoperative day 6 from a primary cesarean section. Blood pressure upon presentation is 178/92. She is admitted for observation and monitoring for preeclampsia.

   Principal/Other Diagnoses_____

3. Patient was recently hospitalized for pneumonia. He was discharged on moxifloxacin. Two days following discharge, he reported onset of diarrhea. The patient was admitted and *Clostridium difficile* antigen came back positive. He also had evidence of acute renal failure due to

CPT only © 2010 American Medical Association. All rights reserved.

dehydration. He was treated with Flagyl p.o. and vigorous hydration and continued treatment for pneumonia.

Principal/Other Diagnoses_____

4. The patient is a newborn baby delivered by cesarean section at 35 weeks for intolerance of labor. Birth weight is 1730 grams. The baby is diagnosed with apnea of prematurity and transient thrombocytopenia.

Principal/Other Diagnoses_____

5. Patient is a 21-month-old male with 1-week history of fever and increased work of breathing. He is admitted, and DFA comes back positive for RSV bronchiolitis. He is given supplemental oxygen and weaned to room air as tolerated. He is also treated for hyponatremia due to dehydration.

Principal/Other Diagnoses_____

6. This female patient is admitted to the hospital for laparoscopic gastric bypass for morbid obesity. She has a body mass index of 53. She also has a history of hypertension, hyperlipidemia, and diabetes.

Principal/Other Diagnoses_____

7. Male patient presents to the emergency room with epistaxis. He thinks he may have accidently taken an extra dose of Coumadin which he takes for atrial fibrillation. Lab results show an abnormal coagulation profile. He is admitted for observation and Coumadin is held. Epistaxis resolves, and he is discharged home in stable condition on regular dose of Coumadin.

Principal/Other Diagnoses_____

8. The patient is admitted to the hospital in acute respiratory failure. She is intubated and maintained on mechanical ventilation. She has a history of congestive heart failure for which she receives Lasix. Patient is diagnosed with acute respiratory failure due to acute systolic heart failure.

Principal/Other Diagnoses_____

9. Mr. Cook presents to the emergency room with 3 days of nausea and vomiting. He is admitted in acute renal failure due to dehydration. He also has a history of end stage renal disease due to diabetic nephropathy and hypertension for which he receives hemodialysis. Acute renal failure resolves with IV hydration. He also receives regularly scheduled hemodialysis while inpatient. Nausea and vomiting are determined due to viral gastroenteritis which resolves on its own.

Principal/Other Diagnoses_____

10. The patient is admitted with chest pain and shortness of breath. Cardiac risk factors include hypertension and hyperlipidemia. The patient is also a smoker. Cardiac catherization shows coronary atherosclerosis. The patient is treated with coronary angioplasty and stent for unstable angina.

Principal/Other Diagnoses_____

## B. Code the following inpatient cases, providing both diagnosis and procedure codes.

1. HISTORY OF PRESENT ILLNESS: The patient is a pleasant 48-year-old female with past medical history significant for hypertension, asthma, and L3–L4 herniated nucleus pulposus. The patient continued to have low back pain as well as right lower extremity radiculopathy and has failed conservative treatment, therefore presents now for further surgical intervention. Current medications are Cardizem and Maxzide inhaler as needed for asthma exacerbation. There are no known allergies.

HOSPITAL COURSE: Following informed consent including risks and benefits of surgical intervention as well as risk stratification by the patient's primary care physician, the patient was brought to the Operating Room, at which time she underwent an L3–L4 lumbar diskectomy. The patient tolerated the procedure well with no complications. The patient during the hospital stay continued to be monitored closely. On postoperative day 1, the patient noted to be hemodynamically and clinically stable and therefore disposition planning was initiated. At the time of dictation, the patient is tolerating a regular p.o. diet, is transitioning to oral pain medication, and will be seen today by Physical Therapy for clearance to home.

FINAL DIAGNOSIS: L3–L4 Herniated Nucleus Pulposus

PRINCIPAL DIAGNOSIS and CODE(S) _____

OTHER DIAGNOSES and CODE(S) _____

PROCEDURE CODE(S) _____

2. HISTORY OF PRESENT ILLNESS: This is a 60-year-old male who was diagnosed with a pituitary adenoma. Past medical history of hypertension and hyperlipidemia. He has no known drug allergies. The patient was consented and scheduled for surgery.

HOSPITAL COURSE: The patient was admitted for transsphenoidal transseptal pituitary tumor resection. The patient remained in the Neurosurgical ICU overnight and remained stable overnight. ENT Team followed him throughout his stay. On postoperative day #1, he was transferred to the regular Neurosurgery Floor where he remained in stable condition and seen by both Physical Therapy and Occupational Therapy Team. On postoperative day #2, the patient was noted to have some swelling in his lips and his left eye, and the Dermatology Team was consulted for possible allergic reaction. They felt that it was not an allergic resection, but it was impetigo. He was placed on doxycycline for a total of 10 days. The patient was discharged home in stable condition.

FINAL DIAGNOSIS: Pituitary Adenoma

PRINCIPAL DIAGNOSIS and CODE(S) _____

OTHER DIAGNOSES and CODE(S) _____

PROCEDURE CODE(S) _____

3. HISTORY OF PRESENT ILLNESS: This is a 23-year-old male who initially presented 6 months ago complaining of double vision, rapidly enlarging right inguinal mass, jaw pain, numb chin, and inability to close the left eye. He had a biopsy of one of his lymph nodes, which was consistent with Burkitt lymphoma. CSF fluid and bone marrow biopsy were both positive for lymphoma. He has since received three cycles of chemotherapy. Most recently, the patient developed some left testicular/groin pain. CT of the abdomen and pelvis showed a 1.4-mm calculus in the left kidney, and this was believed to be the cause of the pain. The patient presents now for cycle 4 of chemotherapy. Surgical history is noncontributory, and he has no known allergies.

HOSPITAL COURSE: This is a 23-year-old male with stage IV Burkitt lymphoma admitted for cycle 4 of chemotherapy. He tolerated the regimen without any complications. The patient's urine was drained during this admission; however, he did not pass any stone despite aggressive hydration that he received with chemotherapy. He was discharged home in stable condition.

FINAL DIAGNOSIS: Burkitt lymphoma

PRINCIPAL DIAGNOSIS and CODE(S) _____

OTHER DIAGNOSES and CODE(S) _____

PROCEDURE CODE(S) _____

4. HISTORY OF PRESENT ILLNESS: The patient is an 81-year-old gentleman, who presents to the Emergency Room from an ECF with a fever of 103. He was complaining of abdominal pain and nausea. His past medical history includes metastatic prostate cancer status post prostatectomy with bony metastatic disease to the lumbar spine, chronic renal insufficiency, with a baseline creatinine of 1.5 to 1.7, history of coronary artery disease, status post pacemaker, hypertension, chronic anemia, and depression. Current medications are Imdur and amlodipine. He is allergic to penicillin.

HOSPITAL COURSE: Fever and leukocytosis: The patient was started on vancomycin and Bactrim for a nosocomial pneumonia. Cultures revealed no growth on his blood cultures × 2 sets, and his urine culture was ultimately mixed flora. The patient defervesced and subsequently had improvement on the vancomycin and the Bactrim.

The vancomycin was discontinued, and the patient was watched on Bactrim alone for 2 days during which time he did not become febrile and additionally clinically remained unchanged.

Acute renal failure: The patient's renal function appeared to have bumped to 2.0 from his baseline of 1.5 to 1.7. He was given IV fluids with subsequent improvement back down to his baseline.

Metastatic prostate cancer: His pain was under fair control; he did respond quite well to the Toradol. However, this was not given on a long-term basis given his underlying chronic kidney disease.

Constipation: The patient appears to have had a history of nausea preventing him from having a good appetite and eating. He reported that he had been having frequent stool which was reported by the exam as well as an abdominal x-ray which showed stool in the colon. He was started on an aggressive bowel regimen with lactulose and Colace. With passing of his bowel movement, the patient's nausea reportedly did improve. The patient also had a CAT scan of his brain to rule out metastasis as a secondary cause for the nausea. The CT was unremarkable.

FINAL DIAGNOSIS: Nosocomial pneumonia

PRINCIPAL DIAGNOSIS and CODE(S) _____

OTHER DIAGNOSES and CODE(S) _____

PROCEDURE CODE(S) _____

5. HISTORY OF PRESENT ILLNESS: This patient is a 29-year-old with intrauterine pregnancy at 38 weeks. The patient was admitted to the hospital stating that she had not had any fetal movement for over 24 hours. The patient was told to come to the hospital immediately for evaluation.

HOSPITAL COURSE: On arrival, the patient was placed on the monitor, was noted to have a deceleration to approximately 90 beats per minute with a recovery followed shortly thereafter by a 2nd deceleration to 60 for another 2 minutes, heart rate then stabilized at 150 for several minutes and deceleration reoccurred. The patient was informed immediately that a cesarean section was necessary. The patient was quickly taken to the Operating Room, and spinal anesthesia was placed without difficulty. Once the heart rate was noted to be approximately 150, the patient was then prepped and draped and underwent a cesarean section. The postoperative course was unremarkable. She was discharged to home on postoperative day #4. The patient is to follow up in 6 weeks.

FINAL DIAGNOSIS: Intrauterine pregnancy with decreased fetal movement

PRINCIPAL DIAGNOSIS and CODE(S) _____

OTHER DIAGNOSES and CODE(S) _____

PROCEDURE CODE(S) _____

6. HISTORY OF PRESENT ILLNESS: The patient is a 75-year-old female who presents for postmenopausal vaginal bleeding. Endometrial biopsy is consistent with endometrial adenocarcinoma. Past medical history of polymyalgia rheumatica, hypertension, thyroid nodules, depression, as well as a right knee replacement. Current medications are Prednisone 5, Hyzaar, Synthroid, and Lexapro.

PHYSICAL EXAMINATION: Vitals are within normal limits. The patient is in no apparent distress. Chest is clear. Heart is regular. Abdomen is soft and benign. Pelvic shows normal vulva, induration of the anterior vaginal wall, suburethral fissures in the small 14-week size nontender uterus. Adnexa are nontender and nonpalpable. Rectal is confirmatory.

HOSPITAL COURSE: The patient was admitted for surgical management of endometrial adenocarcinoma. She underwent laparoscopic vaginal hysterectomy, bilateral salpingo-oophorectomy, pelvic lymph node dissection, and a cystoscopy. Postoperatively, the patient did well. She quickly ambulated and tolerated regular diet and p.o. pain medications. She was given 1 dose of stress dose Solu-Cortef given her history of polymyalgia rheumatica with prednisone use. She was discharged to home on postoperative day #1 in good condition.

FINAL DIAGNOSIS: Endometrial adenocarcinoma

PRINCIPAL DIAGNOSIS and CODE(S) _____

OTHER DIAGNOSES and CODE(S) _____

PROCEDURE CODE(S)_____

7. HISTORY OF PRESENT ILLNESS: This is an 87-year-old woman who presents with a dislodged jejunostomy tube for replacement. The tube was nonfunctioning and missing parts on arrival and draining clear fluid. Therefore, a clamp was placed. Interventional Radiology was consulted and the patient was scheduled for a late afternoon or evening procedure. She was admitted for monitoring for that procedure. Past medical history is significant for diabetes and deep vein thrombosis on lower extremities. She also has a history of a stage IV sacral decubitus ulcer. She has a history of multiple sclerosis with paraplegia, and she is not ambulatory. History of recurrent UTIs, right above knee amputation secondary to nonhealing ulcer and hypertension. She also has hypothyroidism following thyroidectomy and a history of dementia. Current medications consist of Aricept, levothyroxine, a cranberry tablet per J-tube daily, Lopressor, and Coumadin. She is on tube feeds of Jevity every 4 hours.

PHYSICAL EXAMINATION: On admission to the floor, she was afebrile at 97.7, her heart rate was 93, blood pressure 140/78, respiratory rate 18, and saturating 97% on 2 L nasal canula. In general, she is awake and oriented to self. Speaks clearly and appropriately. HEENT exam: Normocephalic and atraumatic. Her pupils 1 mm and minimally reactive to light. Extraocular movements were intact. Her oropharynx looked clear. Her mucous membranes were moist. Her neck showed no lymphadenopathy. It was supple. Full range of motion. Her right eye had a subconjunctival hemorrhage. Cardiac exam was regular rate and rhythm. Pulmonary with clear auscultation anteriorly. Abdomen was soft, nontender, and nondistended. She had good bowel sounds, and the J-tube site was clean, dry, and intact with the tube that was cut and clamped. She has intact sensation in her right AKA. As far as her skin, showed a stage IV 4×2 cm sacral decubitus ulcer that was packed and it had clean margins.

HOSPITAL COURSE: Interventional Radiology was notified that she was scheduled for a placement, which was performed in the evening. We held her Coumadin for 1 dose, but this should be restarted immediately. We had to hold her medications because her J-tube was not functioning, but those were restarted subsequently. Her fingersticks were checked every 6 hours, and she was given normal saline at 75 cc/hour continuously. For her stage IV decubitus ulcer, we did dry-to-dry dressing with Nu Gauze packing and Xeroform and ordered an Eclipse bed for her. She was full code during this hospitalization, and she did very well and had an uneventful J-tube placement. Her tube feeds were restarted, Jevity 1.5 at a goal of 50-cc/hour, and her outpatient medications are unchanged.

FINAL DIAGNOSIS: Jejunostomy tube displacement

PRINCIPAL DIAGNOSIS and CODE(S) _____

OTHER DIAGNOSES and CODE(S) _____

PROCEDURE CODE(S) _____

8. HISTORY OF PRESENT ILLNESS: The patient is an 88-year-old female presenting with an altered mental status. The patient complains of some burning with urination, has been urinating more frequently, and has also decreased appetite. She denies any fevers, night sweats, or chills. She also denies any headache, neck pain, or blurry vision. In the Emergency Department, she was febrile at a temperature of 100.1, pulse of 107, respirations 18, blood pressure 150/79, and saturating 98% on room air. Her past medical history is significant for chronic atrial fibrillation with rate control on Coumadin, congestive heart failure, diastolic dysfunction, mild mitral regurgitation. Other history includes diabetes type 2, hypertension, Paget disease, asthma, and dyslipidemia. Current medications include lisinopril, Lasix, diltiazem, digoxin, warfarin, glipizide, simvastatin, and Protonix. She is allergic to penicillin.

HOSPITAL COURSE: The patient presented to the emergency room with altered mental status, likely in the context of urinary tract infection, and received ceftriaxone. She was also given gentle IV hydration. Blood cultures were obtained as well as urinary culture. Urinary culture grew out Klebsiella also consistent with her urinalysis findings being nitrite negative; therefore, she was continued on ceftriaxone for 3 days IV while in house and will be discharged on 3 additional days of ciprofloxacin 500 mg p.o. b.i.d. Her blood cultures failed to elaborate any evidence of bacteremia. Rate control was achieved parenterally with metoprolol 5 mg IV q.6 hours with her ventricular response rate remaining in the 70 to 80 range. We held her Coumadin overnight. Once she was able to take p.o., we were able to restart her Coumadin as well as the rest of her cardiac medications including lisinopril and Cardizem. Her hyponatremia at the time of admission was initially thought to be secondary to hypovolemic hyponatremia. She was gently rehydrated with isotonic saline, and her sodium improved at the time of discharge. Additionally, for her diabetes, she was covered with sliding scale insulin while n.p.o., and then restarted on her oral hypoglycemics. The remainder of her medical issues remained stable.

FINAL DIAGNOSIS: Klebsiella urinary tract infection

PRINCIPAL DIAGNOSIS and CODE(S) _____

OTHER DIAGNOSES and CODE(S) _____

PROCEDURE CODE(S)_____

9. HISTORY OF PRESENT ILLNESS: This is a 64-year-old gentleman status post fall from a roof approximately 15 feet with positive loss of consciousness. The patient was admitted for management of a right frontal subdural hematoma. The past medical history is significant for obesity, hypertension, diabetes mellitus, and hyperlipidemia. Current medications are actos, glimepiride, lisinopril, aspirin, and simvastatin. There are no known drug allergies.

HOSPITAL COURSE: The patient was admitted to the ICU setting with neurosurgery consult. CT brain was performed. CT brain showed a small subdural hematoma along the medial aspect of the right frontal lobe. Cervical spine showed no acute traumatic injury The patient had a repeat head CT, which showed the small extraaxial hematoma was stable. The patient was transferred out of the ICU setting to the floor. The patient had a right ankle fracture, managed by Orthopedics. Splint was applied. Orthopedics had recommended pain management, elevation of the right lower extremity, nonweightbearing and splint for 4 to 6 weeks. The patient had a right renal subcapsular hematoma. The patient did have some hypertension during his hospital stay as well as some hyperglycemia. The patient was placed on his home medications and Lopressor had been increased. The patient had been placed back on his home medication of lisinopril. Hypertension improved with these medications. The patient was placed back on glimepiride, and the patient had a tight sliding scale regimen, and blood sugars had improved with this. The pain has been well controlled with oral pain medication.

FINAL DIAGNOSIS: Right frontal subdural hematoma, fracture distal tibia/fibula, renal subcasular hematoma

PRINCIPAL DIAGNOSIS and CODE(S) _____

OTHER DIAGNOSES and CODE(S) _____

PROCEDURE CODE(S) _____

10. HISTORY OF PRESENT ILLNESS: The patient is an 83-year-old female who noticed slurring of her speech and an inability to remember people around her. She felt that she had indications of a slight stroke. The patient has had a previous stroke where she feels that she is weak on her right side but feels that these symptoms worsened. The patient's family described that initially the patient was disoriented and did not

seem to be following instructions well but that had cleared up and she seems to be having a hard time getting words out. Her past medical history is significant for old MCA stroke with residual dysphasia and right hemiparesis, hypertension, chronic anemia, and cardiac pacemaker. Current medications include Toprol, Norvasc, and Plavix. The patient has no allergies.

PHYSICAL EXAMINATION: On initial physical exam, her vital signs were heart rate 61, blood pressure 164/75, respiratory rate 22, her oxygen saturation was 100% on room air. In general, she was lying in her bed in no apparent distress. HEENT and Neck Exam: Clear to auscultation. No carotid artery bruits. Cardiovascular: Regular rate and rhythm. No murmurs, rubs, or gallops. Lungs were clear to auscultation bilaterally. Abdominal exam was nontender, nondistended with good bowel sounds. Extremities had no edema. Neurological Exam: Her mental status was alert. She was cooperative. She perseverated. Her repetition was intact. She was able to read 2 words but perseverated on the words. She was not following commands. She was not alert and oriented. Cranial Nerves: Pupils were equal, round, and reactive to light. Extraocular movements were grossly intact. She had a right lower facial droop. Sensation was not tested and hearing was grossly intact. Her motor exam, on the right upper extremity, she was 0/5. She was able to lift her right lower extremity minimally from the bed and she had 5/5 strength in her left upper extremity and left lower extremity. Her sensory exam, she grimaced to nail bed pressure in all four extremities. Coordination and gait were not tested.

HOSPITAL COURSE: The patient is status post left MCA stroke as diagnosed by head CT with worsening aphasia. She was started on aspirin 325 mg daily PR. She had physical and occupational therapy and was evaluated by the speech therapist who recommended home speech therapy at 3 times per week. The patient was found to have greater than 1000 Escherichia coli sent on urinalysis. She was started on Bactrim one double strength tablet q.12 hours.

FINAL DIAGNOSIS: New left MCA stroke with aphasia _____

PRINCIPAL DIAGNOSIS and CODE(S) _____

OTHER DIAGNOSES and CODE(S) _____

PROCEDURE CODE(S) _____

# Coding Quiz: Compliance

NAME _____

_____ 1. Which of the following is *not* required for correctly linked codes?

&#9312; The diagnosis and procedure codes present a logical clinical relationship.
&#9313; The diagnosis and procedures codes are from the same data set.
&#9314; The procedures are necessary and effective, and are not elective or experimental.
&#9315; The treatment is provided at an appropriate level for the presenting problem.

_____ 2. In the diagnostic statement "eye dryness and irritation from insufficient tear production," the primary diagnosis is:

&#9312; eye dryness
&#9313; eye irritation
&#9314; tear production
&#9315; insufficient tear production

_____ 3. The patient presents with transient infiltrations of the lungs by eosinophilia, resulting in cough, fever, and dyspnea. Select the correct diagnosis code(s).

&#9312; 786.2, 780.6
&#9313; 780.6, 786.2
&#9314; 518.3
&#9315; 786.9

_____ 4. Computed tomography without contrast is performed on the maxillofacial area for a patient with chronic sinusitis. Select the correct diagnosis and procedure codes.

&#9312; 473, 70486
&#9313; 473.0, 70486
&#9314; 473.9, 70486
&#9315; 473.8, 70486

_____ 5. An inconclusive diagnosis is indicated by terms such as:

&#9312; rule out, suspected, probable
&#9313; finding, result, report
&#9314; malignant, benign, in situ
&#9315; adverse effect, poisoning, unspecified

_____ 6. Following catheterization and introduction of contrast material, a hysterosonographic study with radiological supervision and interpretation is conducted for a patient with postmenopausal bleeding and suspected endometrial carcinoma. Select the correct diagnosis and procedure codes.

① 239.5, 58350, 76831
② 182.0, 58340, 76831-26
③ 627.1, 58340, 76831-26
④ 627.1, 182.0, 58340, 76831

_____ 7. A biopsy of a dark growth on the back of a patient's hand reported a finding of a 0.9-cm malignant lesion, which was excised under local anesthesia. Select the correct diagnosis and procedure codes.

① 195.4, 17261-47
② 195.4, 17261
③ 709.9, 11621
④ 195.4, 11621

_____ 8. Select the correct codes for an annual physical examination of a 4-year-old established patient.

① V70.0, 99392
② V20.2, 99392
③ V70.0, 99382
④ V70.3, 99401

_____ 9. Following exposure to possible rabies from a dog bite, the patient is inoculated intramuscularly with a rabies vaccine. Choose the correct codes.

① V04.5, E906.0, 90675, 90471
② E906.0, V01.5, 90675, 90471
③ V01.5, E906.0, 90675, 90471
④ V01.5, E906.0, 90675, 90782

_____ 10. Both V codes and E codes may be primary or secondary, depending on the circumstances involved.

① True
② False

_____ 11. Select the correct diagnosis code for the following statement: "The patient suffers from atherosclerotic heart disease caused by plaque deposits in a grafted internal mammary artery. The patient underwent this arterial bypass graft procedure 4 months ago."

① 414.0
② 414.01
③ 414.04
④ 414.9

_____ 12. When the physician owns the equipment and provides the supplies and technical service when providing radiology procedures, the -26 modifier is not appropriate.

① True
② False

_____ 13. After introduction of anesthesia for an intracranial vascular procedure, the patient suddenly went into respiratory distress and the procedure was terminated. What is the correct code?

① 00216-53
② 00216
③ 00210-53
④ 61105-53

_____ 14. In most cases, a biopsy of a site performed with a definitive procedure such as an excision or surgical removal of an organ is not coded.

① True
② False

_____ 15. A patient had a total abdominal hysterectomy 35 days ago and has had increasing pain in the area of the incision. The surgeon performs a diagnostic laparoscopy and, finding adhesions, performs a surgical lysis. Select the correct codes.

① 182.1, 58200
② 614.6, 58660
③ 182.1, 58660-78
④ 614.6, 58660-78

_____ 16. As part of a routine physical examination of a 70-year-old female Medicare patient who sees the doctor every year, the primary care physician orders tests of total serum cholesterol, HDL cholesterol, and triglycerides, and also administers an cytomegalovirus human immune globulin injection. Select the correct codes for the physician's work and the laboratory services.

① V70.0, 99397, G0001, 82465, 83718, 84478, 90291, 90784
② V70.0, 99397, G0001, 80061, 90291, 90784
③ V70.0, 99397, G0001, 36415, J0850, 96372
④ V70.0, 99397, G0001, 80061, 90291, 90781

_____ 17. A patient has a chronic ulcer of the lower limb. During an initial operation, the surgeon prepares the site of the ulcer and uses an allograft to permit healing. Thirty days later, the patient is returned to the OR for a free skin flap. What are the correct codes for the second operation?

① 707.1, 15757
② 707.10, 15757-58
③ 707.8, 15757-59
④ 707.1, 15757-76

_____ 18. A surgeon performs a peritoneoscopy to diagnose reported pain in the right lower quadrant of the patient's abdomen. Based on the findings, the surgeon schedules the patient for a surgical laparoscopic procedure to remove a follicular ovarian cyst. Is the diagnostic procedure included in the surgical procedure in this case?

① Yes
② No

_____ 19. After seeing the patient in the office, the physician admits her for observation. In the hospital, the physician performs a comprehensive history and examination, decision making of high complexity, and decides to schedule the patient for surgery. What procedure code is appropriate?

① 99220
② 99223-57
③ 99291
④ 99220-57

_____ 20. An obstetrician providing routine antepartum, delivery, and postpartum care performs amniocentesis during the first trimester of the patient's pregnancy. Based on CPT, is this service included in the global obstetric package?

① Yes
② No

# Appendixes

## A. ICD-9-CM Official Guidelines for Coding and Reporting Outpatient Services Effective October 1, 2010

### Diagnostic Coding and Reporting Guidelines for Outpatient Services

These coding guidelines for outpatient diagnoses have been approved for use by hospitals/providers in coding and reporting hospital-based outpatient services and provider-based office visits. . . .

The terms *encounter* and *visit* are often used interchangeably in describing outpatient service contacts and, therefore, appear together in these guidelines without distinguishing one from the other.

Though the conventions and general guidelines apply to all settings, coding guidelines for outpatient and providers reporting of diagnoses will vary in a number of instances from those for inpatient diagnoses, recognizing that:

The Uniform Hospital Discharge Data Set (UHDDS) definition of principal diagnosis applies only to inpatients in acute, short-term, long-term care and psychiatric hospitals.

Coding guidelines for inconclusive diagnoses (probable, suspected, rule out, etc.) were developed for inpatient reporting and do not apply to outpatients.

A.  Selection of first-listed condition

   In the outpatient setting, the term first-listed diagnosis is used in lieu of principal diagnosis.

   In determining the first-listed diagnosis the coding conventions of ICD-9-CM, as well as the general and disease specific guidelines take precedence over the outpatient guidelines.

   Diagnoses often are not established at the time of the initial encounter/visit. It may take two or more visits before the diagnosis is confirmed.

   The most critical rule involves beginning the search for the correct code assignment through the Alphabetic Index. Never begin searching initially in the Tabular List as this will lead to coding errors.

1. Outpatient Surgery
   When a patient presents for outpatient surgery, code the reason for the surgery as the first-listed diagnosis (reason for the encounter), even if the surgery is not performed due to a contraindication.

2. Observation Stay
   When a patient is admitted for observation of a medical condition, assign a code for the medical condition as the first-listed diagnosis.
   When a patient presents for outpatient surgery and develops complications requiring admission to observation, code the reason for the surgery as the first reported diagnosis (reason for the encounter), followed by codes for the complications as secondary diagnoses.

B.  The appropriate code or codes from 001.0 through V91.99 must be used to identify diagnoses, symptoms, conditions, problems, complaints, or other reason(s) for the encounter/visit.

C.  For accurate reporting of ICD-9-CM diagnosis codes, the documentation should describe the patient's condition, using terminology which includes specific diagnoses as well as symptoms, problems, or reasons for the encounter. There are ICD-9-CM codes to describe all of these.

D.  The selection of codes 001.0 through 999.9 will frequently be used to describe the reason for the encounter. These codes are from the section of ICD-9-CM for the classification of diseases and injuries (e.g., infectious and parasitic diseases; neoplasms; symptoms, signs, and ill-defined conditions, etc.).

E.  Codes that describe symptoms and signs, as opposed to diagnoses, are acceptable for reporting purposes when a diagnosis has not been established (confirmed) by the provider. Chapter 16 of ICD-9-CM, Symptoms, Signs, and Ill-defined Conditions (codes 780.0–799.9) contains many, but not all, codes for symptoms.

F.  ICD-9-CM provides codes to deal with encounters for circumstances other than a disease or injury. The Supplementary Classification of Factors Influencing Health Status and Contact with Health Services (VO1.0–V89) is provided to deal with occasions when circumstances other than a disease or injury are recorded as diagnosis or problems.

G.  Level of Detail in Coding

    1.  ICD-9-CM is composed of codes with either 3, 4, or 5 digits. Codes with three digits are included in ICD-9-CM as the heading of a category of codes that may be further subdivided by the use of fourth and/or fifth digits, which provide greater specificity.

    2.  A three-digit code is to be used only if it is not further subdivided. Where fourth-digit subcategories and/or fifth-digit subclassifications are provided, they must be assigned. A code is invalid if it has not been coded to the full number of digits required for that code.

H.  List first the ICD-9-CM code for the diagnosis, condition, problem, or other reason for encounter/visit shown in the medical record to be chiefly responsible for the services provided. List additional codes that describe any coexisting conditions. In some cases, the first-listed diagnosis may be a symptom when a diagnosis has not been established (confirmed) by the physician.

I.  Do not code diagnoses documented as "probable," "suspected," "questionable," "rule out," or "working diagnosis." Rather, code the condition(s) to the highest degree of certainty for that encounter/visit, such as symptoms, signs, abnormal test results, or other reason for the visit.

**Please note: This differs from the coding practices used by short-term, acute care, long-term care and psychiatric hospitals.**

J.  Chronic diseases treated on an ongoing basis may be coded and reported as many times as the patient receives treatment and care for the condition(s).

K.  Code all documented conditions that coexist at the time of the encounter/visit, and require or affect patient care treatment or management. Do not code conditions that were previously treated and no longer exist. However, history codes (VIO–V19) may be used as secondary codes if the historical condition or family history has an impact on current care or influences treatment.

L.  For patients receiving diagnostic services only during an encounter/visit, sequence first the diagnosis, condition, problem, or other reason for encounter/visit shown in the medical record to be chiefly responsible for the outpatient services provided during the encounter/visit. Codes for other diagnoses (e.g., chronic conditions) may be sequenced as additional diagnoses.

For encounters for routine laboratory/radiology testing in the absence of any signs, symptoms, or associated diagnosis, assign V72.5 and/or a code from subcategory V72.6. If routine testing is performed during the same encounter as a test to evaluate a sign, symptom, or diagnosis, it is appropriate to assign both the V code and the code describing the reason for the nonroutine test.

For outpatient encounters for diagnostic tests that have been interpreted by a physician, and the final report is available at the time of coding, code any confirmed or definitive diagnosis(es) documented in the interpretation. Do not code related signs and symptoms as additional diagnoses.

**Please note: This differs from the coding practice in the hospital inpatient setting regarding abnormal findings on test results.**

M.  For patients receiving therapeutic services only during an encounter/visit, sequence first the diagnosis, condition, problem, or other reason for encounter/visit shown in the medical record to be chiefly responsible for the outpatient services provided during the encounter/visit. Codes for other diagnoses (e.g., chronic conditions) may be sequenced as additional diagnoses.

The only exception to this rule is that when the primary reason for the admission/encounter is chemotherapy, radiation therapy, or rehabilitation, the appropriate V code for the service is listed first, and the diagnosis or problem for which the service is being performed is listed second.

N.  For patients receiving preoperative evaluations only, sequence first a code from category V72.8, Other specified examinations, to describe the pre-op consultations. Assign a code for the condition to describe the reason for the surgery as an additional diagnosis. Code also any findings related to the pre-op evaluation.

O.  For ambulatory surgery, code the diagnosis for which the surgery was performed. If the postoperative diagnosis is known to be different from the preoperative diagnosis at the time the diagnosis is confirmed, select the postoperative diagnosis for coding, since it is the most definitive.

P.  For routine outpatient prenatal visits when no complications are present, codes V22.0, Supervision of normal first pregnancy, or V22.l, Supervision of other normal pregnancy, should be used as the principal diagnosis. These codes should not be used in conjunction with chapter 11 codes.

# B. CPT Modifiers: Description and Common Use in Main Text Sections

| Code | Description | E/M | Anesthesia | Surgery | Radiology | Pathology | Medicine |
|------|-------------|-----|-----------|---------|-----------|-----------|----------|
| -22 | Increased procedural service | Never | Yes | Yes | Yes | Yes | Yes |
| -23 | Unusual anesthesia | Never | Yes | — | — | — | Never |
| -24 | Unrelated E/M service by the same physician during a postoperative period | Yes | Never | Never | Never | Never | Never |
| -25 | Significant, separately identifiable E/M service by the same physician on the same day of the procedure or other service | Yes | Never | Never | Never | Never | Never |
| -26 | Professional component | — | — | Yes | Yes | Yes | Yes |
| -32 | Mandated services | Yes | Yes | Yes | Yes | Yes | Yes |
| -47 | Anesthesia by surgeon | Never | Never | Yes | Never | Never | Never |
| -50 | Bilateral procedure | — | — | Yes | — | — | — |
| -51 | Multiple procedures | — | Yes | Yes | Yes | Never | Yes |
| -52 | Reduced services | Yes | — | Yes | Yes | Yes | Yes |
| -53 | Discontinued procedure | Never | Yes | Yes | Yes | Yes | Yes |
| -54 | Surgical care only | — | — | Yes | — | — | — |
| -55 | Postoperative management only | — | — | Yes | — | — | Yes |
| -56 | Preoperative management only | — | — | Yes | — | — | Yes |
| -57 | Decision for surgery | Yes | — | — | — | — | Yes |
| -58 | Staged or related procedure/service by the same physician during the postoperative period | — | — | Yes | Yes | — | Yes |
| -59 | Distinct procedural service | — | Yes | Yes | Yes | Yes | Yes |
| -62 | Two surgeons | Never | Never | Yes | Yes | Never | Yes |
| -63 | Procedure performed on Infants | Never | Yes | Yes | Yes | — | Yes |
| -66 | Surgical team | Never | Never | Yes | Yes | Never | — |
| -76 | Repeat procedure by same | — | — | Yes | Yes | — | Yes |
| -77 | Repeat procedure by another physician | — | — | Yes | Yes | — | Yes |
| -78 | Return to the operating room for a related procedure during the postoperative period | — | — | Yes | Yes | — | Yes |
| -79 | Unrelated procedure/service by the same physician during the postoperative period | — | — | Yes | Yes | — | Yes |
| -80 | Assistant surgeon | Never | — | Yes | Yes | — | — |
| -81 | Minimum assistant surgeon | Never | — | Yes | — | — | — |
| -82 | Assistant surgeon (when qualified resident surgeon not available) | Never | — | Yes | — | — | — |
| -90 | Reference (outside) laboratory | — | — | Yes | Yes | Yes | Yes |
| -91 | Repeat clinical diagnostic laboratory test | — | — | Yes | Yes | Yes | Yes |
| -92 | Alternative laboratory platform testing | — | — | Yes | Yes | Yes | Yes |
| -99 | Multiple modifiers | — | — | Yes | Yes | — | Yes |

Key: Yes = commonly used  — = not usually used with the codes in that section
Never = not used with the codes in that section

# CODING QUIZ: ICD-9-CM

| | | | | | | | | |
|---|---|---|---|---|---|---|---|---|
| 1. | ① | ② | ③ | ④ | 21. | ① | ② | ③ | ④ |
| 2. | ① | ② | ③ | ④ | 22. | ① | ② | ③ | ④ |
| 3. | ① | ② | ③ | ④ | 23. | ① | ② | ③ | ④ |
| 4. | ① | ② | ③ | ④ | 24. | ① | ② | ③ | ④ |
| 5. | ① | ② | ③ | ④ | 25. | ① | ② | ③ | ④ |
| 6. | ① | ② | ③ | ④ | 26. | ① | ② | ③ | ④ |
| 7. | ① | ② | ③ | ④ | 27. | ① | ② | ③ | ④ |
| 8. | ① | ② | ③ | ④ | 28. | ① | ② | ③ | ④ |
| 9. | ① | ② | ③ | ④ | 29. | ① | ② | ③ | ④ |
| 10. | ① | ② | ③ | ④ | 30. | ① | ② | ③ | ④ |
| 11. | ① | ② | ③ | ④ | 31. | ① | ② | ③ | ④ |
| 12. | ① | ② | ③ | ④ | 32. | ① | ② | ③ | ④ |
| 13. | ① | ② | ③ | ④ | 33. | ① | ② | ③ | ④ |
| 14. | ① | ② | ③ | ④ | 34. | ① | ② | ③ | ④ |
| 15. | ① | ② | ③ | ④ | 35. | ① | ② | ③ | ④ |
| 16. | ① | ② | ③ | ④ | 36. | ① | ② | ③ | ④ |
| 17. | ① | ② | ③ | ④ | 37. | ① | ② | ③ | ④ |
| 18. | ① | ② | ③ | ④ | 38. | ① | ② | ③ | ④ |
| 19. | ① | ② | ③ | ④ | 39. | ① | ② | ③ | ④ |
| 20. | ① | ② | ③ | ④ | 40. | ① | ② | ③ | ④ |

NAME _____

# CODING QUIZ: CPT and HCPCS

1. ① ② ③ ④          21. ① ② ③ ④
2. ① ② ③ ④          22. ① ② ③ ④
3. ① ② ③ ④          23. ① ② ③ ④
4. ① ② ③ ④          24. ① ② ③ ④
5. ① ② ③ ④          25. ① ② ③ ④
6. ① ② ③ ④          26. ① ② ③ ④
7. ① ② ③ ④          27. ① ② ③ ④
8. ① ② ③ ④          28. ① ② ③ ④
9. ① ② ③ ④          29. ① ② ③ ④
10. ① ② ③ ④          30. ① ② ③ ④
11. ① ② ③ ④          31. ① ② ③ ④
12. ① ② ③ ④          32. ① ② ③ ④
13. ① ② ③ ④          33. ① ② ③ ④
14. ① ② ③ ④          34. ① ② ③ ④
15. ① ② ③ ④          35. ① ② ③ ④
16. ① ② ③ ④          36. ① ② ③ ④
17. ① ② ③ ④          37. ① ② ③ ④
18. ① ② ③ ④          38. ① ② ③ ④
19. ① ② ③ ④          39. ① ② ③ ④
20. ① ② ③ ④          40. ① ② ③ ④

NAME _____

# CODING QUIZ: COMPLIANCE

| | | | | | | | | | |
|---|---|---|---|---|---|---|---|---|---|
| 1. | ① | ② | ③ | ④ | 21. | ① | ② | ③ | ④ |
| 2. | ① | ② | ③ | ④ | 22. | ① | ② | ③ | ④ |
| 3. | ① | ② | ③ | ④ | 23. | ① | ② | ③ | ④ |
| 4. | ① | ② | ③ | ④ | 24. | ① | ② | ③ | ④ |
| 5. | ① | ② | ③ | ④ | 25. | ① | ② | ③ | ④ |
| 6. | ① | ② | ③ | ④ | 26. | ① | ② | ③ | ④ |
| 7. | ① | ② | ③ | ④ | 27. | ① | ② | ③ | ④ |
| 8. | ① | ② | ③ | ④ | 28. | ① | ② | ③ | ④ |
| 9. | ① | ② | ③ | ④ | 29. | ① | ② | ③ | ④ |
| 10. | ① | ② | ③ | ④ | 30. | ① | ② | ③ | ④ |
| 11. | ① | ② | ③ | ④ | 31. | ① | ② | ③ | ④ |
| 12. | ① | ② | ③ | ④ | 32. | ① | ② | ③ | ④ |
| 13. | ① | ② | ③ | ④ | 33. | ① | ② | ③ | ④ |
| 14. | ① | ② | ③ | ④ | 34. | ① | ② | ③ | ④ |
| 15. | ① | ② | ③ | ④ | 35. | ① | ② | ③ | ④ |
| 16. | ① | ② | ③ | ④ | 36. | ① | ② | ③ | ④ |
| 17. | ① | ② | ③ | ④ | 37. | ① | ② | ③ | ④ |
| 18. | ① | ② | ③ | ④ | 38. | ① | ② | ③ | ④ |
| 19. | ① | ② | ③ | ④ | 39. | ① | ② | ③ | ④ |
| 20. | ① | ② | ③ | ④ | 40. | ① | ② | ③ | ④ |

# CODING NOTES

# CODING NOTES

# CODING NOTES

NAME _____

# CODING NOTES